CANCER ETIOLOGY, DIAGNOSIS AND TREATMENTS

BURKITT LYMPHOMA

DIAGNOSIS, RISK FACTORS AND TREATMENT

Cancer Etiology, Diagnosis and Treatments

Additional books and e-books in this series can be found on Nova's website under the Series tab.

CANCER ETIOLOGY, DIAGNOSIS AND TREATMENTS

BURKITT LYMPHOMA

DIAGNOSIS, RISK FACTORS AND TREATMENT

DOUGLAS V. BERTHELOT
EDITOR

nova
Medicine & Health
New York

DOI: https://doi.org/10.52305/VODC3429

Library of Congress Cataloging-in-Publication Data

ISBN: 978-1-68507-071-7

Published by Nova Science Publishers, Inc. † New York

Contents

PREFACE

Burkitt lymphoma (BL) is a form of non-Hodgkin's lymphoma in which cancer starts in immune cells called B-cells. If left untreated, it is rapidly fatal. Chapter one of this monograph evaluates the etiology, pathological issues, diagnosis, clinical manifestations, epidemiology, research, innovation and treatment issues of BL using the clinical systematic review research method and experts' opinion analysis approach. Chapter two reviews the spectrum, unique characteristics and special management considerations when BL develops in specific subgroups of patients with primary immune deficiency disorders. Chapter three reviews the incidence, clinicopathological and epidemiologic features, treatment and outcome data available in pediatric and adult patients with post solid organ transplant BL. Chapter four focuses on the pathobiology and the treatment of first-line and relapsed/refractory cases of BL and describes new therapeutic strategies which could improve results in this pathology. Chapter five examines the therapeutic advances in BL and its variants. Finally, Chapter six explores and emphasizes the trends and issues in research and innovation in the characteristics, clinical updates and management approaches of BL.

Chapter 1 - Burkitt lymphoma is a rarely encountered aggressive non-Hodgkin B-cell lymphoma. The disease is associated with Epstein Barr virus, human immunodeficiency virus, and chromosomal translocations that cause the overexpression of oncogene C-MYC. Although the critical role of MYC in Burkitt's lymphoma has been well described, recent biological insights have identified several new mutations that cooperate with MYC in driving lymphomagenesis, paving the way for novel drug testing in this disease. The World Health Organization classifies Burkitt lymphoma into three clinical groups: endemic, sporadic and immunodeficiency-related. The endemic form is linked to malaria and Epstein Barr virus. The immunodeficiency-related variant is associated with human immunodeficiency virus and to a lesser extent, organ transplantation. With intense chemotherapy treatment disease prognosis is excellent in children but poor in adults. In addition, recently, intermediate-intensity approaches have been tested in Burkitt lymphoma. Early multicenter results demonstrate good tolerability while maintaining high cure rates in all patient and age groups. There is a need for more awareness of the trends and issues surrounding the diagnosis and treatment of Burkitt lymphoma. Hence the purpose of this chapter is to evaluate the etiology, pathological issues, diagnosis, clinical manifestations, epidemiology, research and innovation and treatment issues of Burkitt lymphoma using clinical systematic review research method, and experts' opinion analysis approach.

Chapter 2 - Mature B cell Non-Hodgkin lymphoma (B-NHL) including Burkitt lymphoma (BL) and diffuse large B cell lymphoma (DLBCL) are among the most common malignancies associated with primary immune deficiency disorders (PIDs). Unlike sporadic BL, PIDs associated B-NHL are commonly Epstein Barr virus (EBV) driven. There is a wide spectrum of PIDs associated with BL resulting in unique features with each association. For example, patients with X-linked lymphoproliferative disease type 1 (XLP1) are at particularly high risk of developing multiple lymphomas. Other PIDs are also chromosome instability syndromes, such as ataxia telangiectasia (AT) and Bloom Syndrome (BS). In these syndromes, chemotherapy, if not modified, confers a high risk of severe morbidity and mortality. Patients with PIDs are routinely excluded from clinical trials of B-NHL, therefore, limited data are available regarding potential differences in lymphoma biology, risk factors, optimal treatment strategies, and outcome. The prognosis of these patients is overall poor due to increased treatment-related toxicities and/or treatment refractoriness. These patients require modifications of certain components of intensive therapy with careful attention to supportive care, but there is no consensus with regard to the optimal treatment strategies. Historically, many patients with PIDs associated lymphomas were treated with minimal or modified reduced-intensity therapy. The incorporation of novel targeted agents like monoclonal antibodies into less intensive standard chemotherapy regimens may help address the challenges of treatment-associated toxicities and refractory disease. Immunotherapies, however, bring uncertainties of the quality and duration of subsequent immune reconstitution. Despite the rarity of these cases, every pediatric and lymphoma oncologist will face these challenges in their career. After 3 real world case presentations, this chapter will review the spectrum, unique characteristics and special management considerations when BL develops in specific subgroups of patients with PIDs.

Chapter 3 - The incidence of Burkitt lymphoma (BL) is markedly elevated in solid organ transplant recipients compared to the general population. It is frequently a late event occurring more than 1-2 years after transplantation. This in contrast to other forms of post-transplant lymphoproliferative disorders (PTLD), the majority of which occur in the first year after transplantation. Post solid organ transplant Burkitt lymphoma (PSOT-BL) is most often Epstein Barr virus (EBV) positive, in contrast to sporadic BL (sBL) in immunocompetent patients (IC-BL). It differs from other forms of monomorphic post-transplant lymphoproliferative disorders (M-PTLD) with a distinct pathologic and molecular profile. There is no defined standard treatment regimen for PSOT-BL and both adult and pediatric studies have used approaches ranging from low dose chemotherapy regimens with or without the addition of rituximab to more intensive immunochemotherapeutic regimens similar to those used for IC-BL. The latter approach appears to be more effective, though treatment related morbidity and mortality remain major limitations, particularly in older patients. Of particular concern are the risk of infection related death, risk of rejection and higher risk of end organ toxicities specific to the allograft. Guidelines for treatment modification and data on the impact on survival, graft function or long-term toxicity are lacking. In this chapter the authors will review the incidence, clinicopathological and epidemiologic features, treatment and outcome data available in pediatric and adult patients with PSOT-BL. Finally the authors will focus on specific treatment considerations and the unique challenges in designing regimens based on the organ transplanted and patient comorbidities.

Chapter 4 - Burkitt lymphoma (BL) is an uncommon mature B cell non-Hodgkin lymphoma (NHL) characterized by aggressive clinical behavior with high survival rates among children and young adults. Three different variants are well recognized which differ in epidemiology, clinical presentation, and molecular or biological features. Endemic, sporadic and immunodeficiency-associated are these BL epidemiological forms. The genetic hallmark is the rearrangement of the MYC oncogene, virtually presented in all BL cases. Translocation with the immunoglobulin heavy chain gene region, t(8;14)(q24;q32), is the most frequent (80%). Recently, promising findings by RNA sequencing studies have expanded the molecular landscape with the identification of novel genes probably involved in its pathogenesis. Mutations in the transcription factor TCF3 or ID3 (its negative regulator) have been described in endemic, sporadic, and immunodeficiency-associated BL. Clinical presentation differs according to the epidemiologic variants with nodal and extranodal involvement (central nervous system, bone marrow, gastrointestinal tract). Tumor lysis syndrome, before or after treatment, is frequent because of the massive proliferation rate of BL, being mandatory an appropriate prophylaxis. Initial chemotherapy approaches were based on acute lymphoblastic leukemia intensive pediatrics regimens showing high efficacy in young patients while significant toxicity in older and immunocompromised patients. Addition of anti CD20 therapy to chemotherapy improved previous outcomes becoming the standard of care in BL. Optimize chemotherapy regimens to decrease toxicity, relapsed/refractory approaches, and incorporate biological findings on treatment are the main goal of the new era of BL management. In this chapter, the authors will describe the main aspects of this entity, focusing on the pathobiology and the treatment both, in the first-line and relapsed/refractory cases, besides describing the new therapeutic strategies, which in the long term, could improve the results in this pathology.

Chapter 5 - Burkitt lymphomas are aggressive B-cell cancers (non-Hodgkin type of lymphomas) that frequently involve aggressive progression in the bone marrow and in the central nervous system. Burkitt lymphoma (also known as small non-cleaved cell lymphoma and Burkitt's lymphoma) has a variant termed Burkitt-like lymphoma or BLL. Other types or Burkitt lymphomas are termed: Endemic or African is a type that usually involves the jaw and the facial bones; Sporadic Burkitt lymphoma involves abdominal tumors and Immunodeficiency-related Burkitt lymphoma has lymph node and bone marrow involvement. The World Health Organization suggests that there is little difference between Burkitt lymphoma and BLL and considers them essentially the same disease. The order variants are classified under the term Burkitt lymphoma. Due to their rapid progression, these lymphomas are considered medical emergencies that require fast diagnosis and efficient treatment. Hence this clinical systematic review and experts' opinions analyses examines the therapeutic advances in Burkitt lymphoma.

Chapter 6 - Burkitt lymphoma is an uncommon but highly aggressive B-cell Non-Hodgkin Lymphoma. It is a subtype of mature B-cell lymphoma and can be treated successfully within a short period via high-intensity chemotherapeutic regimens. Diagnosis and initial workup must be completed rapidly to begin treatment due to high proliferation of the disease. Burkitt lymphoma is associated with the Epstein-Barr Virus and with chromosomal translocation that activates the c-MYC gene. However, by implementing chemotherapy regimens, complete remission and overall survival for young patients with BL remains high. In contrast, in elderly patients and those with relapsed/refractory disease, the prognosis remains a medical challenge. Rituximab has been shown to improve patient survival rate. However, because resistance can still occur, further treatment and evaluation is required, including inhibition of the MYC proto-oncogene through the use of bromodomain inhibitors. In this clinical systematic review and experts' opinions analysis, the authors explore and emphasise the trends and issues in research and innovation in the characteristics, clinical updates and management approaches of Burkitt lymphoma.

In: Burkitt Lymphoma
Editor: Douglas V. Berthelot

ISBN: 978-1-68507-071-7

Chapter 1

BURKITT LYMPHOMA: DIAGNOSIS AND TREATMENT ISSUES

Daniella E.C.C.O.H Kingsley-Godwin*, MD, PhD, Maria Jana Kingsley Godwin and Joshua Kingsley-Godwin, PhD

London Medical Academy, London, England, United Kingdom

ABSTRACT

Burkitt lymphoma is a rarely encountered aggressive non-Hodgkin B-cell lymphoma. The disease is associated with Epstein Barr virus, human immunodeficiency virus, and chromosomal translocations that cause the overexpression of oncogene C-MYC. Although the critical role of MYC in Burkitt's lymphoma has been well described, recent biological insights have identified several new mutations that cooperate with MYC in driving lymphomagenesis, paving the way for novel drug testing in this disease. The World Health Organization classifies Burkitt lymphoma into three clinical groups: endemic, sporadic and immunodeficiency-related. The endemic form is linked to malaria and Epstein Barr virus. The immunodeficiency-related variant is associated with human

* Corresponding Author's E-mail: daniellagodwin@ymail.com; dkingsley@iahcp.uk.

immunodeficiency virus and to a lesser extent, organ transplantation. With intense chemotherapy treatment disease prognosis is excellent in children but poor in adults. In addition, recently, intermediate-intensity approaches have been tested in Burkitt lymphoma. Early multicenter results demonstrate good tolerability while maintaining high cure rates in all patient and age groups. There is a need for more awareness of the trends and issues surrounding the diagnosis and treatment of Burkitt lymphoma. Hence the purpose of this chapter is to evaluate the etiology, pathological issues, diagnosis, clinical manifestations, epidemiology, research and innovation and treatment issues of Burkitt lymphoma using clinical systematic review research method, and experts' opinion analysis approach.

Keywords: Burkitt, lymphoma, Burkitt's, diagnosis, risk factors, epidemiology, treatment, lymphomagenesis, global, etiology, pathogenesis, prognosis, research, MYC, C-MYC, lymphatic, lymphoid, Epstein-Barr virus, EBV

INTRODUCTION

Lymphoma is any of a group of malignant diseases of the lymphatic system that usually starts in the lymph nodes or in lymphoid tissues of other organs, such as the lungs, spleen, skin etc. Lymphomas are generally classified into two types: Hodgkin disease (HD) or Hodgkin's lymphoma (HL) and non-Hodgkin lymphoma (NHL) [1]. Hodgkin disease results in enlargement of the lymph nodes and spleen. As HD generally has a high cure rate, non-Hodgkin lymphomas are often more difficult to treat and manage in some cases. Burkitt lymphoma (BL) is a form of non-Hodgkin's lymphoma in which cancer starts in immune cells called B-cells, which affects primarily the upper and lower jaws, orbit, retroperitoneal tissues situated near the pancreas, kidneys, ovaries, testes, thyroid, adrenal glands, heart, and pleura, that occurs especially in children of central Africa area, and that is associated with Epstein-Barr virus (EBV) [1-3].

BL is named after the British Surgeon, Denis Burkitt, who first identified this unusual disease in 1956 among children in Africa [3]. In Africa, BL is common in young children who also have malaria and EBV, the virus that causes infectious mononucleosis. One mechanism may be that malaria weakens the immune system's response to EBV, allowing it to change infected B-cells into cancerous cells. It has been reported that about 98% of African cases are associated with EBV infection [2, 3].

Outside of Africa, BL is rare. For example, in the United States of America (USA), about 1,200 people are diagnosed each year with BL, and about 59% of the diagnosed patients are over age 40 [2, 3]. It has been indicated that BL is especially likely to develop in people infected with human immunodeficiency virus (HIV), the virus that causes acquired immunodeficiency syndrome (AIDS) [3]. Before highly active antiretroviral therapy (HAART) became a widespread treatment for HIV/AIDS, the incidence of BL was estimated to be 1,000 times higher in HIV-positive people than in the general population [2-4]. A form known as endemic BL is the most common childhood cancer in Africa, where the disease was discovered [3, 4], which research suggests that it may be linked in some way to the EBV [1-5] as stated above.

Other NHLs are referred to in a number of ways that describe the morphology of the cells and whether the tumors are diffuse or nodular [4, 5]. Overall, the nodular type of disease progresses more slowly than the diffuse type [2, 4, 5]. Diffuse large-cell lymphomas are more aggressive and can involve the liver, the lungs, the kidneys, and even the brain [2, 4, 6]. Some lymphomas invade the bloodstream, causing leukemia [3-6]. Diagnosis of either major forms of lymphoma, including BL requires laboratory analysis of tissues, usually from the lymph nodes [1, 2, 6].

Known as a fast growing human tumor, BL is associated with impaired immunity and is rapidly fatal if left untreated [1-8]. However, intensive chemotherapy can achieve long-term survival in more than half the people with BL [1, 3-8]. The purpose of this chapter is to evaluate the etiology, pathological issues, diagnosis, clinical manifestations, epidemiology, research and innovation and treatment issues of Burkitt lymphoma using clinical systematic review research method, and experts' opinion analysis approach.

METHODS

A clinical systematic review research method and experts' opinions analysis approach were used in carrying out this study in order to track down and analyze all materials that deal with the diagnosis, treatment and epidemiology of BL, including other healthcare issues associated with it globally. To this end, we performed a systematic review and search of all articles and publications, including other materials published and unpublished describing the clinical manifestations, pathological issues, diagnosis, treatment and epidemiology of BL internationally. Experts' opinions reports were also searched for, obtained and included in the study.

A search was also conducted in online and electronic databases like PubMed/Medline, EMBASE, SCOPUS etc., using the terms: "Burkitt lymphoma, diagnosis, risk factors, epidemiology, treatment, lymphomagenesis and global" to track down all data/information from April 1948 to April 2021. Only articles and materials published in English language, and reporting on data collected internationally between April 1948 and April 2021 were included in the study.

Reference lists of review studies and articles included in the review were screened for titles that included the key terms.

Inclusion Criteria

Studies, articles, publications, various materials and experts' opinions reports were included if they met the following inclusion criteria:

1) Published in English language in the period between April 1948 and April 2021 with a full text available.
2) The studies or projects and experts' opinions reports are original in nature, and the articles, publications and materials are well written for the targeted audience and purpose.

3) Predominantly focusing on the etiology, types/classifications, clinical manifestations, diagnosis, treatment and epidemiology of BL.
4) Predominantly focusing on BL, not on the more general lymphoma topics
5) Focusing on the population as a whole, not only on a specific subgroup (for example, farmers, elderly, adults, students, children, etc.)
6) Study or project period should be at least one year in duration.
7) Only including data from April 1948 or later that addressed the issues under investigation.
8) Not only focusing on mild symptoms of BL
9) If multiple publications used the same study population, the most recent report was used, as it generally addressed a larger population.

Data Extraction

Relevant papers, projects and experts' reports were selected by screening the retrieved articles, publications and reports through the database searches thus:

- the titles (first step)
- abstracts/report summaries (second step)
- entire articles, publications and reports (third step)

The same process was also used in the library catalogue searches for relevant publications, books, theses, including searches from governmental, medical and healthcare facilities that dealt with the matters under evaluation.

During each step, the title, abstract/summary or entire article or publication was screened to ensure that it met the inclusion criteria. This screening was conducted by all the authors independently. Extracted data included source population, study period, study group size, case ascertainment, case criteria, incidence, age distribution, sex distribution, mortality and most frequent cause of BL, the clinical presentations, diagnosis, treatment, healthcare issues, research and innovations and overall management strategies of the disease.

Methodological Quality

Characteristics and methodological quality of selected studies, reports and publications were evaluated with a particular focus on study design, case ascertainment, case definition, patient population and the description of the methodology, including sources of data and the information contained in the other publications.

In the relevant data, we based the evaluation of methodological quality on five elements of the STROBE checklist [9, 10] which were most relevant to the quality of reported epidemiology (incidence and mortality rates): study design, setting, participants, data sources/measurement, study size etc.

In addition, quality of data presented under clinical manifestations, pathophysiology, histopathology, diagnosis, staging, treatment, management, patient evaluation, complications, healthcare matters, research and innovations etc., were also evaluated.

Data and Statistical Analysis

Statistical analysis including averages and checking of percentages were done using EXCEL for Windows version 2010 where and when applicable in order to confirm the accuracy of reported data/information that we have stated in this article.

RESULTS

The systematic search of articles and publications, including all materials published and unpublished describing the diagnosis, treatment and epidemiology of BL globally, and healthcare issues linked to it, plus experts opinions report analysis from April 1948 to April 2021 yielded the following data:

- The Online Databases search from PubMed, EMBASE, SCOPUS and other databases identified 2,593 articles
- All other published materials in BL in journals, books, grey literature identified 405 materials
- Unpublished materials such as projects on BL academic theses for PhD studies and Masters' degrees and general information on BL etc., identified 103 materials.

In total, 3,101 articles and publications, including all materials published and unpublished describing the diagnosis, treatment and epidemiology of BL globally were identified, as stated in points I to iii above.

Two hundred and thirty five (235) duplicates were removed, resulting in 2,866 potentially relevant articles, citations and publications. Following the screening of titles, abstracts and the critical review of the entire articles and publications, a total of 100 articles and publications were retained for inclusion in this systematic review (Figure 1).

The classification, etiology, staging, clinical manifestations, pathological issues, diagnosis, treatment and epidemiology of BL globally, including multi-professional healthcare team management need and research and innovations in the diagnosis and treatment advances of BL are described and discussed in the sections below.

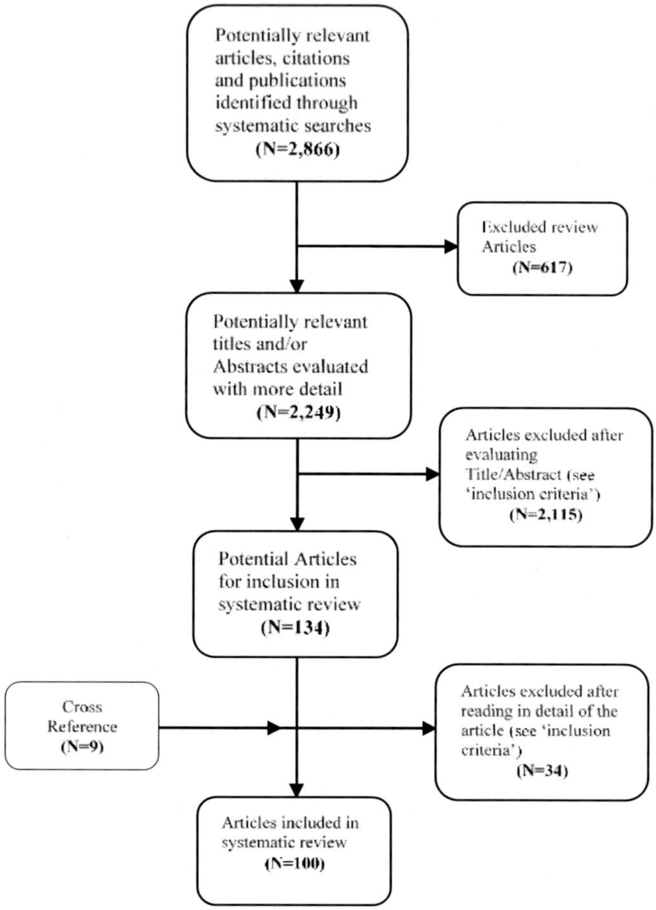

Figure 1. Flow Chart of the Literature Search and selection of articles and publications used for the study.

Classification of Burkitt Lymphoma

BL can be divided into three main clinical variants or types: the endemic, the sporadic, and the immunodefiency-associated variants. The descriptions of each type are stated as follows [2, 3, 13]:

The Endemic Type (Which Is Also Known as "African Variant")

This type most commonly occurs in children living in malaria endemic regions of the world (for example, equatorial Africa, Brazil and Papua New Guinea) [2, 4, 11]. EBV infection is found in nearly all patients [2, 9, 11]. Chronic malaria is believed to reduce resistance to EBV, allowing it to take hold. The disease characteristically involves the jaw or other facial bone, distal ileum, cecum, ovaries, kidney and breast.

The Sporadic Type of BL (Also Known as "Non-African" Variant)

This is the most common variant found in places where malaria is not holoendemic. The tumor cells have a similar appearance to the cancer cells of classical endemic BL. Sporadic lymphomas are rarely associated with EBV [12], NHL, which includes BL, accounts for 30-50% of childhood lymphoma [2, 12]. The jaw is less commonly involved, compared to the endemic variant. The ileocecal region is the common site of involvement [3, 10-12].

Immunodeficiency-Associated BL

This is usually associated with HIV infection [13] or occurs in the setting of post-transplant patients who are taking immunosuppressive drugs. BL can be one of the diseases associated with the initial manifestation of AIDS [11-13].

It is difficult to differentiate between these three clinical variants/types morphologically by their microscopic appearance or by their immunophenotype. Immunodeficiency-linked BL may demonstrate more plasmacytic appearance or more pleomorphism, but these features are not specific.

BL is commonly associated with the infection of B cell lymphocytes with the EBV and in these cases, it is considered to be one form of the EBV associated lymphoproliferative disease. The epidemic variant of BL (eBL) is in almost all cases associated with EBV infection [14].

On the other hand, the sporadic variant, which afflicts ~ 1,200 individuals/year in the US [14], is associated with the virus in only 10-15% of cases [2, 15].

The immunodeficiency-associated variant of BL affects 30-40% of people with HIV-induced AIDS [4, 15] and rare cases of patients who received a bone marrow or other organ transplant: in the latter cases, patients have certainly received intensive chemotherapy and therefore are immunodeficient [2, 15]. About 30% of people with the immunodeficiency variant are infected with EBV [16].

The fact that some BL cases do not involve EBV shows that many cases of the disease are not caused by EBV, which means that the virus may be an innocent passenger organism in these cases. However, the almost ubiquitous presence of the virus in the epidemic variant of BL suggests that it contributes to the development and/or progression of this variant [17] in this case. The mutational landscape in BL has recently been found to differ between tumors with and without EBV infection, indicating further strengthening the role of the virus in lymphomagenesis [6, 17].

Etiology of BL

BL is associated with EBV. The exact mechanism underlying EBV and B-cell malignancy remains unclear. Epstein-Barr nuclear antigen 1 (EBNA1) protein is an EBV latent protein expressed in endemic BL [2, 17]. EBNA2 gene deletion leads to the expression of EBNA3 genes (i.e., EBNA3A-C). Tumor cells derived from these cell lines are resistant to apoptosis; thus, EBNA2 might confer a survival advantage for the neoplastic cells.

BL is endemic to areas where malaria is holoendemic, such as Brazil, Papua New Guinea, and equatorial Africa. It has been reported that there is a direct correlation between endemic BL and increased Plasmodium falciparum antibody titers [2, 17].

Immunodeficiency-associated BL is linked to HIV. On the contrary, the incidence of lymphoma is higher when the patient has a CD4 count greater than 200 and no opportunistic infection. It is not clear how HIV affects the risk of endemic BL [2, 17].

Symptoms of BL

The symptoms of BL depend on the type. The endemic (African) variant usually starts as tumors of the jaw or other facial bones [2, 3, 17]. It also can affect the gastrointestinal tract, ovaries, and breasts and can spread to the central nervous system, causing nerve damage, weakness, and paralysis [2, 3, 13, 17].

Sporadic and immunodeficiency-associated types of BL more commonly seen in the United States of America (USA), and they usually start in the bowel and form a bulky tumor mass in the abdomen, often with massive involvement of the liver, spleen, and bone marrow [2, 13, 15-17]. These variants can also start in the ovaries, testes, or other organs, and spread to the brain and spinal fluid [3, 13, 15, 17].

Other symptoms associated with BL include loss of appetite, weight loss, fatigue, night sweats and unexplained fever [12-17].

Epidemiology of BL

Amongst all cancers involving the same class of blood cell, 2.3% of cases are BL [18], and EBV infection is strongly correlated with this cancer [19].

BL accounts for approximately 1% to 5% of all NHLs [20]. BL is more common in Caucasians than people of African or Asian descent. As with most types of lymphoma, BL is more prevalent in males with a 3-4:1 male-to-female ratio [21]. The distribution of endemic cases of BL in Africa and Papua New Guinea corresponds to areas where malaria and EBV are prevalent [18, 21]. In children younger than 18 years of age, the incidence is approximately 3 to 6 cases per 100,000 children annually [2, 18, 21]. The average age of diagnosis is six years [19, 21].

The sporadic form is localized to North America and Europe with a median age of diagnosis of 45 [19-21]. Sporadic BL has an annual estimated incidence of 4 per 1 million children less than 16 years of age whereas the incidence is 2.5 per 1 million in adults [18, 20-21]. The average age of diagnosis in pediatric patients is three to 12 years of age. The immunodeficiency-associated variant has an incidence of 22 per 100,000 persons in die United States [20, 21].

Epidemiologic Features of Endemic, Sporadic and AIDS-Associated BL

The epidemiologic pertinent features of the three different types of BL are outlined in Table 1 below [3, 21].

Table 1. Three epidemiologically distinct forms of Burkitt lymphoma (BL) [22]

Form of BL	Geographic location	Incidence, per 100,000/y	% EBV association	Cofactors
Endemic*	Equatorial Africa and Papua New Guinea	5-10, for age 3-12 y	100	Holoendemic malaria
Sporadic†	Worldwide, varies with location	10- to100-fold less than e-BL	15-85	Not clearly established
AIDS-assoc‡	Worldwide, data from untreated HIV carriers	10- to 100-fold more than e-BL	30-40	HIV

Key to Symbols Used in Table 1:

*Endemic BL (e-BL) occurs where Plasmodium falciparum malaria is holoendemic; incidence rates from African data.

†Values for sporadic BL incidence and EBV association vary with location worldwide. In Northern Europe and the U.S., the disease occurs with 100-fold lower incidence than e-BL, and 15–20% tumors are EBV^+. In some other areas (North Africa, North Brazil) incidence is only 10-fold lower than e-BL, and 85% of tumors are EBV^+.

‡Values are based on data from untreated AIDS cohorts in the early years of the AIDS epidemic in the U.S. and Europe.

The summary of epidemiologic issues in this section is as follows [22]:

- The high-incidence "endemic" form typically presents as a jaw or abdominal tumor in children in areas of equatorial Africa and Papua New Guinea, where malaria is holoendemic, and is 100% EBV genome–positive.

- Elsewhere BL occurs in "sporadic" form, again mainly in children, at intermediate to low incidence and with different degrees of EBV association depending upon the area.
- Western countries show the lowest incidence rates and the weakest virus association, with only 15% to 20% tumors being EBV positive ($^{+}$); by contrast, BL appears to be more common in other locations, for example, equatorial areas of Brazil, and EBV-association rates are correspondingly higher.
- It is therefore possible that chronic immune stimulation from other parasitic infections may also increase BL incidence to some degree and that this increase also preferentially involves EBV-associated disease.
- Remarkably, a third, adult form of the tumor, AIDS-BL, proved to be very common among HIV-infected individuals, often appearing as one of the first symptoms of AIDS; 30% to 40% of these tumors carry EBV.
- Significantly, all BLs, irrespective of form or EBV status, carry a reciprocal translocation that places the c-myc gene under the control of either the heavy- or light-chain immunoglobulin (IgH or IgL) loci, leading to high-level c-myc expression. Such c-myc deregulation therefore appears to be the obligatory defining feature of BL pathogenesis, often with EBV acting as a complementary oncogenic agent, and other infections such as malaria or HIV, though not oncogenic *per se*, somehow accentuating lymphoma risk.

Pathophysiology

BL originates from germinal center B cells [13, 23]. The c-myc gene is involved in the pathogenesis of BL [5, 13, 23]. The MYC family is composed of regulator genes and oncogenes that encode transcription factors that regulate the cell cycle [5, 23]. Translocations of the c-myc gene on chromosome 8 are the hallmark of BL, occurring in approximately 95%

of cases [2, 21, 23]. The t(8;14)(q24;q32) is the most common translocation in BL, occurring in 70% to 80% [21, 23]. The MYC oncogene is relocated to be juxtaposed to the promoter sequence of the immunoglobulin IgG heavy chain (IgH) gene leading to constitutive activation of MYC [5, 21, 23]. Other translocations include t(2;8Xpl2; q24) and t(8;22)(q24; q11) [2, 5, 21, 23]. The collocation of the MYC oncogene to the heavy chain (14q32), kappa light chain (2p12) or lambda light chain (22q11) of the immunoglobulin gene results in the dysregulation of the MYC. The presence of an MYC rearrangement is not specific for BL [5, 23].

In addition to the characteristic translocation of c-myc, many gene mutations have been identified, including truncating mutations of ARID1A, amplification of MCLI, truncating alterations of PTEN, NOTCH, and ATM; amplifications of RAF1, MDM2, KRAS, 1KBKE, deletion of CDKN2A, and CCND3 activating mutations [5, 6, 21-23]. In normal B-cells, MYC overexpression causes apoptosis via a p53-dependent pathway [23]. In the neoplastic cells of BL, it is not uncommon for tumor suppressor gene TP53 to be mutated [6, 21, 23].

In endemic BL, EBV latent proteins prevent apoptosis in B-cells containing the c-myc translocation via EBNA1 protein, BHRF1 protein, EBER transcripts, vIL-10, BZLF1, and LMPl [5, 6, 23]. The prevention of apoptosis likely gives rise to the malignant clone of B-cells [5, 23]. EBV is implicated in promoting genomic instability, telomere dysfunction, and DNA damage [19, 23].

Plasmodium falciparum prompts the reactivation of latent EBV [5, 19, 21-23]. In addition, P. falciparum can activate toll-like receptor 9 (TLR9) which induces immunoglobulin-MYC translocations [3, 5, 23]. Cytidine deaminase allows for B-cells to switch from IgM expression to the expression of other immunoglobulin subtypes [5, 23]. Aberrant expression of cytidine deaminase is correlated with c-myc translocation [5, 17, 23]. The enzyme is not detected in HIV- positive patients that do not have Burkitt lymphoma [5, 15, 23].

The genetic dimension, the role of MicroRNA expression, BL Pathogenesis and EBV manifestation and the roles of holoendemic malaria and HIV infection in BL pathogenesis are described below:

Genetics

All types of BL are characterized by dysregulation of the ***c***-myc gene by one of three chromosomal translocations [24]. This gene is found at 8q24 [6, 24]. The following points are also noted:

- The most common variant is t(8;14)(q24;q32), which accounts for about 85% [24] of cases. This involves c-myc and IGH@ [6, 23-25]. A variant of this, a three-way translocation, (8; 14; 18), has also been identified [25].
- A rare variant is at t(2;8)(pl2;q24) [26]. This involves IGK@ and c-myc [25, 26].
- Another rare variant is t(8;22)(q24;ql 1) [26]. This involves IGL@ and c-myc [25, 26].

The two less-common translocations: t(2;8)(pl2;q24) and t(8;22)(q24;ql 1), account for the remaining 15% of cases not due to the t(8;14)(q24;q32) translocation [6, 24, 26].

MicroRNA Expression

It was described that short non-coding RNAs named microRNAs (miRNAs) have important functions in lymphoma biology [24-26]. In malignant B cells, miRNAs participate in pathways fundamental to B cell development, like B cell receptor (BCR) signaling, B cell migration/adhesion, cell-cell interactions in immune niches, and the production and class- switching of immunoglobulins [24-26].

BL Pathogenesis and EBV Manifestation

Despite the fact that EBV is a gamma1-herpesvirus carried by the vast majority of people worldwide as a lifelong asymptomatic infection, it has growth-transforming potential and it is also etiologically linked to a variety of B-cell, T/NK-cell and epithelial malignancies [15-17, 27]. Indeed the use of the full growth-transforming program appears to be restricted to B cells and, in essence, infecting such cells *in vitro* leads to the outgrowth of permanent EBV^+ lymphoblastoid cell lines (LCLs) [27]. This growth-transforming program (called Latency III) involves expression of six EB nuclear antigens—EBNAs 1, 2, 3A, 3B, 3C and -LP—from one of two adjacent promoters Wp or Cp and two latent membrane proteins—LMPs 1 and 2—from their own promoters [17, 27]. Additionally, *Bam*HIA rightward transcripts (BARTS, a presumed source of the virally encoded *Bam*HIA microRNAs) and the non-coding EBER transcripts are detectable here, as well as in all other forms of latency [26, 27]. This same program is also seen in most cases of EBV-driven post-transplantation lymphoproliferative disease (PTLD) lesions to which immunosuppressed patients who have received transplants are particularly prone [27, 28].

On the other hand, EBV^+ BLs (whether endemic, sporadic or AIDS-associated) typically display more restricted forms of latency; in effect, it is clear from *in vitro* models that the full Latency III program is incompatible with the high-level c-myc expression that is the essential determinant of the BL phenotype [29]. Hence, most BLs carry EBV as a Latency I infection, with the genome maintenance protein EBNA1 being expressed from an alternative promoter Qp, in addition to the BARTS and non-coding EBER transcripts [15-17, 28, 29]. More recently, a subset of 3 from 20 endemic BL tumors have been identified that display a Wp-restricted form of EBV latency where, in addition to the BARTS and EBER transcripts, EBNAs1, 3A, 3B, 3C and -LP are expressed from the Wp promoter; these tumors are distinct in carrying a mutant form of the viral genome with a deletion of the EBNA2 gene, such that EBNA2 and the EBNA2-induced LMP proteins are not expressed. Importantly, this form of restricted viral latency also appears to be compatible with the c-myc–driven growth program [6, 15-17, 27-29].

In the past decades, a project team, Kelly and Rickinson [30] identified an endemic tumor which, though homogeneous for the t(8:14) translocation and other genetic changes, was nevertheless heterogeneous at the single-cell level with respect to EBV infection [15-17, 29, 30]. This tumor, called Awia-BL, yielded multiple subclones *in vitro,* some of which showed Latency I infection, others Wp-restricted latency, and others a novel "EBNA2$^+$, LMP1$^-$" latency characterized by expression of all six EBNAs again in the absence of LMPs; once again, all three types of subclone retained typically high c-myc levels and a BL-like cellular phenotype [31].

The frequency of EBV's association with BL (particularly endemic BL), and the fact that all EBV$^+$ BLs (whether endemic, sporadic or AIDS-associated) carry the virus in every cell of the malignant clone, implies a definitive role for the virus in tumor pathogenesis, but the nature of that role has long remained in doubt [26, 27, 29-31]. Hints that the virus might complement the deregulated c-myc gene by acting as an anti-apoptotic rather than as a growth-promoting agent first came from work with an EBV$^+$ sporadic tumor, Akata-BL, which is unusual in that it generates rare EBV-genome–negative cells in late passage [32].

Comparison of EBV$^+$ and EBV$^-$ Akata-BL clones revealed that a Latency I EBV infection provided the cells with a slight, but significant, protection from apoptotic triggers [29, 31-33]. Similar observations have since been seen with rare endemic BL lines yielding EBV-loss subclones in late passage [33] and now more importantly from an early passage tumor [31, 33]. The mechanism of protection mediated by Latency I infection, and indeed the viral gene product responsible, remains a contested issue [33-36].

In contrast, Wp-restricted latency was found to provide much stronger protection from apoptosis [35-38], perhaps explaining why this form of infection is represented relatively frequently in endemic BL (vis-à-vis Latency I) despite its establishment being dependent on the very rare circumstance of infection with an EBNA2 gene–deleted virus [36-38]. Very interestingly, recent work has shown that Wp-restricted tumors are distinguished from Latency I BLs in showing greatly reduced expression of the pro-apoptotic Bcl2 family protein, Bim [39] (Kelly et al, manuscript in preparation). This therefore provides a conceptual link between EBV's postulated role as an anti-apoptotic agent in BL pathogenesis and the work in murine models identifying uncoupling of the c-myc/Bim connection as a key factor in lymphomagenesis driven by mutant c-myc alleles [15-17, 35, 38, 39].

It will however be interesting to determine whether endemic BLs with Wp-restricted latency are more likely than Latency I tumors to carry a wild-type c-myc allele. This would be consistent with the hypothesis that one or more of the additional viral gene products expressed in Wp-restricted tumors actively downregulate Bim and could therefore substitute for the effects of c-myc mutation [30, 31, 35-39].

The Roles of Holoendemic Malaria and HIV Infection in BL Pathogenesis

The potentially important insights into tumor pathogenesis that could come from studying the other predisposing infections such as:

- the widely accepted role of holoendemic *Plasmodium falciparum* malaria as the environmental factor underlying the 100-fold higher incidence of endemic BL (all EBV^+) compared with that of the sporadic tumor in Western societies [19, 33-39].
- the even more dramatic increase in BL incidence (both EBV^+ and EBV^- disease) seen in individuals infected by HIV are sometimes overlooked in BL discussions [39-41].

It is firstly important to note that AIDS-BL is not a product of profound immune impairment but typically arises as an early symptom of AIDS at a time when patients still retain T-cell competence and display persistent lymphadenopathy rather than lymphodepletion [39-41]. Furthermore, early work on HIV-associated lymphadopathy lesions clearly showed highly expanded germinal center activity [40, 41], consistent with expansion of the very stage of B-cell differentiation where c-myc translocation and subsequent mutation would be most anticipated. The heightened risk of BL imposed by HIV is therefore most likely due to the still poorly understood ability of this virus to activate the B-cell system [5, 41]. Interestingly, the EBV load in circulating B cells is also elevated to a new steady-state level in the early years following primary HIV infection, and this again appears to be linked to direct effects upon the B-cell system and not to any detectable impairment of EBV-specific T-cell surveillance [33-39, 41].

Likewise, malaria is known to provide a chronic stimulus to the B-cell system, and several recent studies have shown that EBV loads are remarkably high in African children generally, and in children with malaria in particular [42, 43]. It remains to be seen to what extent holoendemic malaria's role as a cofactor in BL development reflects its global B-cell stimulatory capacity intrinsically, and to what extent its gross disturbance of the EBV-host balance is mediated either as a byproduct of the above stimulation or by other mechanisms (reviewed in Rochford et al) [44]. In this latter context, there is preliminary evidence of an inhibitory effect of acute malaria on EBV-specific T-cell surveillance [45]. However, there is stronger evidence that the cysteine-rich interdomain region 1α (CIDR1α) of the malaria protein *P falciparum* erythrocyte membrane protein 1 (PfEMP1), expressed at the surface of parasitized red blood cells can activate B cells, in particular the memory B-cell pool in which EBV persists [46, 47]. This could have the dual effect of expanding the pool of latently infected cells *in vivo* and, by inducing the reactivation of some infected cells into EBV lytic cycle [48], of increasing total EBV loads. These various possibilities are not mutually exclusive. The triple strand of malarial infection, EBV-host balance and BL risk indeed has been established as basis for current and future projects, with the ability to reveal new insights into BL pathogenesis, diagnosis, treatment and long term management. [15-17, 33-39, 47].

Histopathology

BL is an aggressive B-cell lymphoma comprising a monomorphic population of intermediatesized mature lymphocytes [2, 3, 25, 48]. The cells contain round nuclei with lacy chromatin and may have one or more small nucleoli [25, 48]. The cells characteristically have basophilic cytoplasm with prominent vacuoles [7, 25, 48].

On hematoxylin-eosin (HandE) stained sections, the cells have distinct cytoplasmic borders giving them a molded appearance (Figure 2) [26, 48]. Morphological variants are plasmacytoid or pleomorphic [2, 3, 26, 48]. The neoplastic cells are highly proliferative, which is reflected in the increased number of mitotic figures. Increased cell turnover is countered by increased apoptosis. In tissue, this results in a "starry sky" appearance due to tingible-body macrophages containing cellular debris as can be seen in Figure 2 [2, 26, 48].

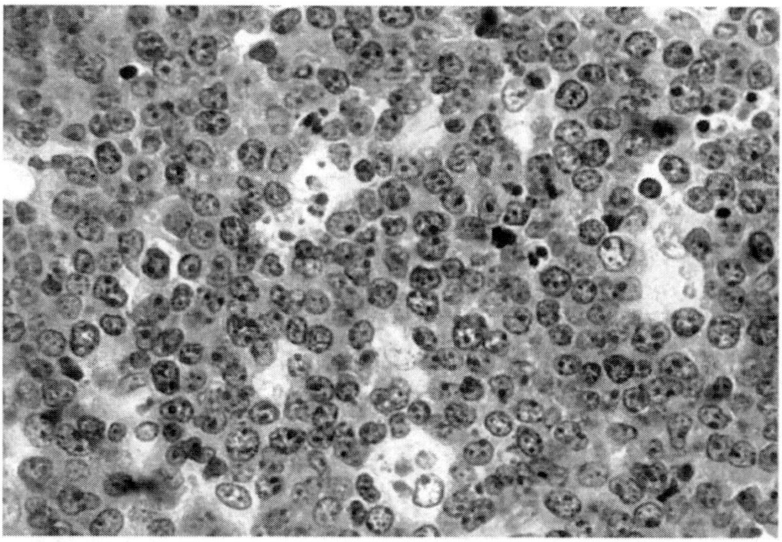

Figure 2. The tumour cells of B lymphoblasts which are large rounded or indented nucleus and 3 or 4 nucleoli with thin layer of basophilic cytoplasm are closely opposed to each other forming a dark blue background (the 'sky'). The surrounding macrophages with abundant pale foamy cytoplasm scattered among the tumour cells (the stars) [26, 48].

In other words, the various types of BL show a typical histological feature, with a malignant population of round monomorphic B cells, interspersed with macrophages that give the tumor histology a "starry sky" pattern, as can be seen in figure 2 [26, 48].

Immunohistochemistry and cytogenetics play a significant role in the diagnosis and management of BL [24-26, 48]. The malignant B-cells express surface IgM. The cells are positive for B-cell markers including CD 19, CD20, CD79a, and PAX5 [24-26]. They are positive for germinal center markers CD 10 and bcl-6 but are negative for bcl-2 [25, 26, 48]. The neoplastic cells do not express T-cell markers and do not express immature markers TdT or CD34. Rapid cell turnover is reflected by high Ki67 positivity nearing 100%, which is a very helpful diagnostic clue [2, 7, 24-26, 48].

Patient History and Physical Examination

Patients with BL often present with a rapidly growing mass, elevated lactate dehydrogenase (LDH), and increased uric acid levels because of the tumor's rapid doubling time [3, 23, 126]. The primary site of sporadic BL is typically the abdomen, but the head and neck may be affected as well [2, 23, 26, 48].

Patients also present with abdominal pain secondary to ileocecal disease, abdominal distention, nausea, vomiting, and gastrointestinal bleeding [2, 3, 14, 48]. Adult patients are more likely to present with constitutional symptoms like fever, weight loss, night sweats [14, 20, 48].

Occasionally, patients have jaw or bone marrow involvement. BL rarely involves the mediastinum, central nervous system, testes, skin, thyroid gland, and breast [2, 14, 20, 48] Endemic BL characteristically presents with an enlarging jaw lesion, periorbital swelling, or genitourinary involvement (Figure 3) [49]. Jaw involvement is seen predominantly in children [3, 21, 22, 49].

Malnourishment is common at disease presentation [3, 49]. If the patient has bone marrow involvement consisting of greater than 25% of cellularity, then the disease is classified as BL [28, 49]. A purely leukemic presentation is rare [2, 3, 49].

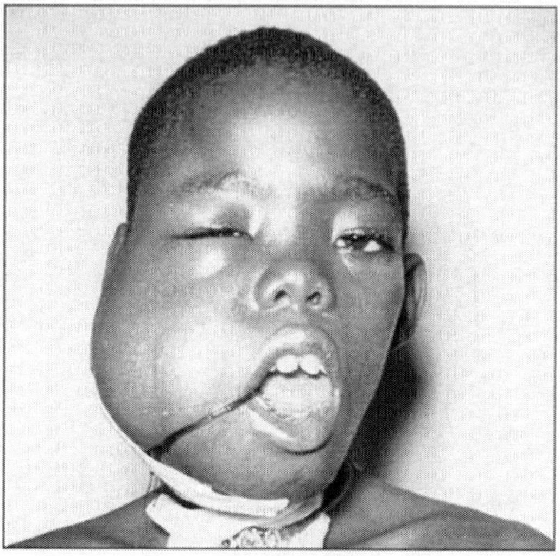

Figure 3. Clinical photograph shows a large tumor of the mandible in an African boy [3, 6, 27, 49].

Diagnosis of BL

As BL spreads so quickly, prompt diagnosis is essential in order to achieve efficient patient care [2, 3, 50]. If BL is suspected, all or part of an enlarged lymph node or other suspicious disease site will be biopsied, and a sample of tissue is examined under a microscope. This will confirm or rule out BL [49, 50].

Other diagnostic features and matters are described and discussed below [26-52].

Characteristics/Features of Malignant B Cells

Normal B cells of a germinal center possess rearranged immunoglobulin heavy and light chain genes, and each isolated B cell possesses a unique IgH gene rearrangement [26, 50-52]. Since BL and other B-cell lymphomas are a clonal 50, 52]. When the DNA of tumor cells is analyzed using electrophoresis, a clonal band can be demonstrated, since identical IgH genes will move to the same position [26, 50, 52].

On the contrary, when a normal or reactive lymph node is analyzed using the same technique, a smear rather than a distinct band will be seen [50, 52]. This technique is useful since sometimes benign reactive processes, for example, infectious mononucleosis, and malignant lymphoma can be difficult to differentiate [50-52].

Microscopic Investigations

The tumor consists of sheets of a monotonous (i.e., similar in size and morphology) population of medium-sized lymphoid cells with high proliferative and apoptotic activity. The "starry sky" appearance seen [26, 48, 49, 51, 52] under low power (Figure 2) is due to scattered tingible body-laden macrophages (macrophages containing dead apoptotic tumor cells). It has been asserted that the old descriptive term of "small non-cleaved cell" is misleading [26, 49-52]. The tumor cells are mostly medium in size (i.e., tumor nuclei size similar to that of histiocytes or endothelial cells). "Small non-cleaved cells" are compared to "large non-cleaved cells" of normal germinal center lymphocytes [26-52]. Tumor cells possess small amounts of basophilic cytoplasm with three to tour small nucleoli [49, 52]. The cellular outline usually appears squared off [49, 52].

Immunohistochemistry Analysis

The tumor cells in BL generally strongly express markers of B cell differentiation (CD20, CD22, CD 19), as well as CD 10 and BCL6. The tumor cells are generally negative for BCL2 and TdT [49, 52].

The high mitotic activity of BL is confirmed by nearly 100% of the cells staining positive for Ki67 [52].

Additional tests to be undertaken may include [16-22, 52]:

- Computed tomographic (CT) imaging of the chest, abdomen, and pelvis
- Chest X-ray
- Positron emission tomography (PET) or gallium scan
- Bone marrow biopsy
- Spinal fluid examination via lumbar picture procedure

- Biochemistry blood tests to measure kidney and liver functions
- Testing for HIV disease

Evaluation and Laboratory Tests for Patients

Obtaining adequate tissue is paramount to the diagnosis of BL [7, 52]. Fine-needle aspiration might not provide enough tissue for the diagnosis, and as result, excisional biopsy is preferred. Superficial lymph node or pleural fluid may be sampled for diagnosis. In developed countries, BL is suspected by microscopy or flow cytometry and confirmed by immunohistochemistry and cytogenetics [2, 52]. In medical centers without access to confirmatory testing facilities, the diagnosis of BL may be made with by fine-needle aspiration and clinical correlation of events [2, 3, 52].

After a tissue diagnosis is made, bone marrow aspiration and biopsy, as well as cerebrospinal fluid (CSF) evaluation should be undertaken in order to determine the extent of involvement of the tissue [51, 52]. CT scans of the chest, abdomen, and pelvis are firstly undertaken [14, 52]. Whole body PET and CT scans should be done but this should not delay treatment [2, 51, 52].

Essential required laboratory tests include [2, 51, 52]:

- Complete blood count (CBC)/Full blood count (FBC) with differential
- Erythrocyte sedimentation rate (ESR)
- Complete metabolic panel (CMP) such as:
    - prothrombin time (PT)
    - partial thromboplastin time (PTT)
    - serum lactate dehydrogenase
    - uric acid
    - hepatitis B serology
    - pregnancy testing in women
- HIV testing

In areas with limited resources, ultrasonography may aid in the staging of the disease [8, 52].

Staging of BL

If a person is diagnosed with cancer, his/her clinician will inform him/her what stage the cancer is at based on various factors, which will also describe the size of the tumor/cancer, and how far it has spread. Cancer is typically labeled in stages from I to IV, with IV being the most serious one. Those broad groups are based on a much more detailed system that includes specific information about the tumor and how it affects the rest of the body. Thus the stage of a tumor is the extent to which it has spread in the body. Unfortunately, different project groups/teams have different ways of staging BL. For example, the St. Jude staging system is routinely used for pediatric patients, whereas the Ann Arbor system and Murphy staging system are commonly used for adults. The Ann Arbor system accounts for the patient's symptoms. The Murphy staging system is used because of its emphasis on extranodal disease, and for distinguishing bone marrow involvement from central nervous system disease.

Due to the aggressive nature of BL in adult patients, staging should be performed using bone marrow, and lumbar puncture samples and treatment started immediately after confirmation of diagnosis [2, 3, 14, 52].

The descriptions of the St. Jude and Ann Arbor staging systems are outlined below:

St. Jude/Murphy Staging System in Children

The stages of the St. Jude/Murphy Staging System in Children are described below [2, 7, 52, 53]:

Stage I

This consists of a single tumor (extranodal) or a single anatomical area (nodal), excluding mediastinum or abdomen or a tumor (extranodal) with regional node involvement, on the same side of the diaphragm.

Stage II

This involves a single tumour (extranodal) with regional node involvement, lymph node involvement on same side of the diaphragm (two or more nodal areas or two single extranodal tumors, with or without regional node involvement), or a primary gastrointestinal tract tumour (usually ileocecal) with or without associated mesenteric node involvement, grossly completely resected.

Stage III

This occurs on both sides of the diaphragm (two or more nodal areas or two single extranodal tumors), all primary intrathoracic tumors (for example, mediastinal or pleural thymic), all extensive primary intraabdominal disease; unresectable abdominal disease, even if only in one area, or all primary paraspinal or epidural tumors, irrespective of other sites.

Stage IV

This includes any of the above stages (I to III) with initial CNS or bone marrow involvement (only if less than 25% of the marrow is composed of Burkitt cells).

The Murphy Staging System in Adults

The Murphy Staging System in adults is described below [2, 7, 51-53]:

Stage I

This involves single nodal or extranodal site excluding the mediastinum or abdomen.

Stage II

This consists of two or more nodal areas on one side of the diaphragm.

Stage HR (Hormone Receptor Stage)

This refers to completely resectable abdominal disease stage.

Stage III

This involves two or more nodal areas on opposite sides of the diaphragm, or a primary intrathoracic tumor, paraspinal or epidural tumors, extensive intra-abdominal disease.

Stage III A

This is a completely non-resectable abdominal disease.

Stage III B

Widespread multiorgan intra-abdominal disease.

Stage IV

Central nervous system or bone marrow involvement Favorable: Stage I or HR [7, 51, 52].

Ann Arbor System in Adult

Stage I

This involves a single nodal or extranodal site.

Stage II

This comprises of two or more nodal areas on one side of the diaphragm, or localized involvement of an extra-lymphatic site and one or more sites on the same side of the diaphragm (IIE).

Stage III

This involves two or more nodal areas on opposite sides of the diaphragm which may include/ involvement of the spleen (IIIs), or localized involvement of an extranodal site (HIE).

Stage IV

This consists of diffuse or disseminated involvement of one or more extra-lymphatic sites, or two single extranodal tumors on opposite sides of the diaphragm.

Please note that the favorable stages for patients are: Stages I, II and III [7, 52].

In summary, a staging system is a standard way for the cancer care team to describe how far a cancer has spread. Hence, a lymphoma's stage is the extent of the disease at the time of diagnosis. The treatment and prognosis (outlook) for a child with an NHL depend, to a large extent, on the lymphoma's stage. The stage is based on the results of physical exams, biopsies, and imaging tests (CT scan, PET scan, etc.), which have been discussed and described in the sections of patient history and physical examination, diagnosis and patient evaluation above. The staging system most often used to describe the spread of NHL in children is called the *St. Jude staging system.* This is different from the staging system used for lymphomas in adults, which is called the Ann Abor system, as described above.

Differential Diagnosis

The differential diagnosis of BL primarily includes other CD 10 positive B-cell lymphomas [7, 52]:

- diffuse large B-cell lymphoma (DLBCL)
- high-grade follicular lymphoma
- B-cell acute lymphoblastic leukemia/lymphoma (B-ALL).

Both DLBCL and high-grade follicular lymphoma typically have larger cells with more pleomorphism than is expected with BL. BCL2 positivity and a Ki67 proliferation index less than 90% favor a diagnosis other than BL [52]. Finding an MYC translocation is not diagnostic of BL; approximately 10% of DLBCL have an MYC translocation [5, 7, 30, 52]. B-ALL may resemble BL in size, but it typically has finer chromatin. By immunohistochemistry or flow cytometry, B- ALL will often express markers of immaturity such as CD34 and/or TdT [51, 52].

There are also some uncommonly encountered entities to consider. Cases with BL-type morphology that lack an MYC translocation should be examined for abnormalities of chromosome 11q for the diagnosis of "Burkitt-like lymphoma with 11q aberration" [5, 7, 29, 52]. The prognosis for this recently described entity appears similar to BL [29, 30, 52].

Therefore, a diagnosis of BL begins with a good medical history and physical examination. The diagnosis of BL is usually confirmed with tumor biopsy. The involvement of the bone marrow and central nervous system are usually remarkable. The spread of the cancer can determined and achieved by the analysis of bone marrow and spinal fluid.

The involvement of lymph node and organ can be used in the staging of BL as described above. Hence stage IV can be confirmed by the involvement of bone marrow or the central nervous system. Confirmation of the involvement of the organs or lymph nodes can be done via CT scan or MRI scan as described in the evaluation section.

Risk Factors for BL

BL is most likely to affect children [2, 3, 21, 30, 52] and it is uncommon in adults [2, 14, 19-21, 52]. The disease is more common in males and people with compromised immune systems, like those who have HIV. The incidence of BL is higher in certain regions such as [2, 21, 52, 53]:

- North Africa
- Middle East
- South America
- Papua New Guinea

Sporadic and endemic forms of BL are associated with EBV [2, 3, 53]. It has also been indicated that insect-borne viral infections and herbal extracts that promote tumor growth are possible contributing factors [21, 52, 53].

Treatment and Management Issues

It has been recommended that treatment for BL should begin promptly, at least within 48 hours of diagnosis without being delayed for further studies [53, 54].

In developed countries, the overall cure rate for sporadic BL approaches 90% in pediatric and young adult populations [29, 52-54]. Treatment is stratified based on patient's age and stage. In pediatric patients with complete surgical resection of disease, it is recommended that patients receive two cycles of chemotherapy of moderate-intensity like cyclophosphamide, vincristine, prednisolone, and doxorubicin [6, 21, 22, 54].

In pediatric patients with stage I and II disease, overall survival is greater than 98% [2, 21, 22, 25, 52, 54]. For children with residual or stage III disease, it is advised that the patient receives a minimum of four cycles of dose-intensive chemotherapy, for example, two cycles of cyclophosphamide, vincristine, prednisolone, doxorubicin and high-dose methotrexate [21, 22, 25, 52, 54]. After this, the patient should receive two cycles of cytarabine and high-dose methotrexate [3, 6, 21, 22, 54]. Intrathecal therapy is administered concurrently with chemotherapy [22, 54].

Furthermore, in pediatric patients with CNS or bone marrow involvement, it is recommended that patients receive up to eight cycles of dose-intensive chemotherapy (i.e., two cycles of cyclophosphamide, vincristine, prednisolone, doxorubicin, and high-dose methotrexate) plus two courses of cytarabine and etoposide, in addition to four courses of maintenance chemotherapy (i.e., vincristine, prednisolone, high-dose methotrexate, cyclophosphamide, doxorubicin, cytarabine, and etoposide) [6, 21, 22, 54]. Like residual or stage ΠI disease, intrathecal therapy is administered concomitantly with chemotherapy [55-57].

Standard chemotherapy regimens, such as cyclophosphamide, doxorubicin, vincristine, and prednisone (CHOP) are inadequate in treating adult BL [14, 20, 55-57]. Current recommendations are offered by the

National Comprehensive Cancer Network and include multiagent regimens with CNS prophylaxis [53-57]:

- R-hyper-CVAD [54]
- CODOX-M/IVACA [55] with or without rituximab [56]
- dose-adjusted EPOCH with rituximab [57]

Immunotherapy has a role in treatment. Rituximab (anti-CD20) should be a component of all treatment regimens as it is correlated with a positive prognosis [55-57]. Newer anti-CD20 agents, of atumumab and obinutuzumab, are under investigation. Blinatumomab, an Anti-CD 19 monoclonal antibody, and inotuzumab, an anti-CD22 monoclonal antibody, are under investigation [20, 55-57]. Experimental drugs to inhibit the growth of BL B-cells by inducing apoptosis include histone acetylase inhibitors such as rapamycin, valproic acid and tubacin, and mTOR inhibitors like temsirolimus [14, 20, 54-57]. Anti-PD1 agents prevent tumor cells from evading the immune system via the PD1 pathway. Therapies inhibiting the MYC oncogene are under investigation [5, 20, 21, 57].

Highly active anti-retroviral therapy (HARRT) has allowed for the management of immunodeficiency-related BL using high dose chemotherapy in patients with HIV [56, 57]. In this patient population, it is advised that less toxic chemotherapy is used because of the susceptibility to organ failure and infection [7, 57].

In patients with relapsing disease, the prognosis is typically poor, and treatment will depend on the specific clinical scenario [14, 20, 55, 57]. However, the development of more effective chemotherapy drugs (i.e., ifosfamide, carboplatin, etoposide) is improving patient outcomes. Salvage regimens may include R-IVAC, R-GDP, R-ICE, DHAP [21, 57]. Autologous and allogeneic hematopoietic cell transplant may be considered [58]. In elderly patients who cannot endure intense chemotherapy, treatment is often palliative [14, 20, 55, 58].

As described above in this section, in general, the first line of treatment for BL is intensive chemotherapy [54-58]. A few of these regimens are: the GMALL-B-ALL/NHL2002 protocol, the modified Magrath regimen (R-

CODOX-M/IVAC) [59]. COPADM [60], hyper-CVAD [61], and the Cancer and Leukemia Group B (CALGB) 8811 regimen [62]; these can be associated withrituximab [62, 63]. In older patients treatment may be dose-adjusted EPOCH with rituximab [64].

The effects of the chemotherapy, as with all cancers, depend on the time of diagnosis. With faster-growing cancers, such as BL, the cancer actually responds faster than with slower-growing cancers [53-58, 64]. This rapid response to chemotherapy can be hazardous to the patient, as a phenomenon called "tumor lysis syndrome" could occur [21, 62, 65]. Close monitoring of the patient adequate hydration is essential during the process [62, 65]. Since BL has high propensity to spread to the central nervous system, for example, lymphomatous meningitis, intrathecal chemotherapy with methotrexate and/or ARA-C and/or prednisolone is given along with systemic chemotherapy [55-57, 65].

Examples of some chemotherapy include cyclophosphamide, doxorubicin, vincristine, methotrexate, cytarabine, ifosfamide, etoposide and rituximab [65].

Other treatments for BL include immunotherapy, bone marrow transplants, stem cell transplant, surgery to remove the tumor and radiotherapy [64, 65].

Toxicity and Side Effect Management

Tumor lysis syndrome, which is the cytolysis of tumor cells causing hyperuricemia, hyperkalemia, hyperphosphatemia, and hypocalcemia, is often a consequence of high proliferative rates seen in Burkitt lymphoma and may also be provoked by chemotherapy [21, 65]. Calcium can precipitate in the kidneys, causing acute kidney injury (AKI) [21, 22, 65]. The flux of calcium, phosphate, and potassium is associated with cardiac arrhythmias, CNS toxicity, and death [14, 20, 55, 58, 65]. As TLS can occur before treatment is initiated, prophylaxis should be started promptly [55-58, 65]. Tumor lysis syndrome is more likely to occur in male patients, as well as patients with a history of renal disease, elevated lactate dehydrogenase (LDH) or uric acid levels, or splenomegaly [21, 57, 62, 65]. Rigorous hydration before and after chemotherapy treatment, allopurinol and rasburicase have improved patient's outcomes [20, 21, 22, 54, 58, 65]. Hemodialysis is advised if the patient develops severe kidney injury [20, 21, 22, 54, 58, 65].

Chemotherapy is associated with significant side effects, namely hematologic toxicity and severe infection risk. In underdeveloped nations, treatment must be catered to account for socioeconomic factors [2, 65]. Supportive care is essential, particularly the prevention of tumor lysis syndrome, fever management, and nutrition supplementation. Due to the high cost, lack of access to medical care, and health illiteracy many patients do not complete the recommended treatment. In patients with endemic BL, 1-year event-free survival is a gauge of long-term survival (risk of relapse is less than or equal to 5% after 1 year) [2, 3, 20, 21, 22, 55, 65].

Complications of BL

The complications of BL depend on the type and stage of the lymphoma, and the nature of the treatment used in the management of the disease. Patients could have short- and long-term problems from the tumor or from treatment side effects, and these may include issues such as [65, 66]:

- Enhanced risk for infection
- Enhanced risk for bleeding
- Feeling of nausea and vomiting
- Issues with diarrhea
- Malnutrition and poor appetite
- Mouth sores
- Loss of hair
- Cardiovascular disease
- Pulmonary issues

- Possibility of developing other cancers in the future
- Infertility issues Trouble having children (infertility)

Side effects on various chemotherapies can be treated in order to get them under control. Effective patient education would help in preventing anxieties and worries from patients and their families.

Prognosis of BL

Prognosis of BL is dependent on clinical and histopathological staging, particularly the extent of disease. In general, younger patients have a better prognosis [59, 61, 66]. Therefore, it is possible that pediatric patients are better able to tolerate intense chemotherapy [21, 22, 59, 61, 66].

Poor response to cyclophosphamide, prednisolone, and vincristine are poor prognostic indicators, as well as detection of CNS disease at presentation [20, 55, 58, 66]. Elevated lactose dehydrogenase concentrations (twice the upper limit of normal values) is associated with poor outcomes [55, 58, 66]. The finding of some additional cytogenetic findings beyond the MYC translocation, including deletion of 13q, a gain of 7q, or complex cytogenetics may portend a worse prognosis [21, 63, 65, 66].

Double hit mutations in ID3, CCND3, and mutations in 18q21 CN-LOH indicate a poor response to therapy and poor prognosis [65, 66]. Malnourishment, particularly in low-income countries, is associated with neutropenia secondary to chemotherapy [2, 3, 54, 55, 57, 59, 66].

In immunodeficiency-related BL, low CD4 count is a poor prognostic indicator [60, 66]. When BL relapses within six months of treatment completion, the prognosis is poor because of the limited availability of new drugs for treatment as most were exhausted during initial therapy [55-57, 60, 65, 66].

Conversely, in developing nations where treatment is less aggressive, a greater number of children can be treated after relapse [59, 61].

In developing countries, the stage of the disease and abdominal ultrasound are used to determine prognosis [2, 3, 52, 66]. Fluorodeoxyglucose positron emission tomography (PET) scans are utilized to evaluate for residual or recurrent disease [52, 65, 66]. The prognostic significance of early PET scans or CT scans to assess disease is an area of investigation [52, 65, 66]. Research is being conducted to explain whether minimal residual disease (MRD) is a risk factor for worse prognosis in BL [65, 66]. Polymerase chain reaction (PCR) can be used to assess MRD by detecting MYC/IgH fusion [5, 29, 66].

Therefore the patient outcome depends on the stage of BL at diagnosis. It has been noted that the outlook is usually worse in adults over the age of 40, but treatment for adults has improved in recent years [64-66]. The outlook is poor in people who have HIV, but it is significantly better in people whose cancer has not spread to other parts of the body [60, 65, 66].

Multi-Professional Healthcare Team Management Need

The diagnosis, evaluation, treatment and management of BL require a team of healthcare providers comprising at least; a pathologist, hematologist, oncologist, pharmacist, nurse and radiologist, plus the help of other healthcare professionals in order to achieve prompt diagnosis and administer treatments as quickly as possible for achieving better outcomes for patients. When there is suspicion for BL, communication between team members is critical to providing quick diagnosis with judicious use of ancillary tests such as FISH for MYC translocations [5, 29, 64, 66].

Research and Innovations in the Diagnosis and Treatment Advances of BL

In recent years, there have been some research and innovative projects in the diagnosis and treatments advances of BL, some of the recent research projects are stated below.

Research in Diagnostic Advances of BL

Some of the research trends and issues in the diagnostic advances of BL are described and discussed below:

Gene Targets

Unique genetic alterations promote cell survival in BL, which is different from other types of lymphomas [67]. These *TCF3* and ID3 gene mutations in BL correspond to a cell survival pathway that may be found to be amenable to targeted therapy [68].

Issues in BL Pathogenesis and Cellular Genetic Change

BL pathogenesis and cellular genetic change is considered as highly aggressive B cell neoplasm characterized by the translocation and deregulation of the MYC gene on chromosome 8. Six distinct clinical changes of BL are described and discussed below.

The Effects of C-Myc Overexpression and C-Myc Translocation

C-myc is a transcription factor involved in many cellular processes including growth, proliferation and apoptosis [5, 29, 69]. In accordance with this global role, c-myc expression is tightly regulated and immediately sensitive to external stimuli. In normal cells, c-myc's pro-proliferative effects, exemplified by upregulation of cyclins D and E and down-regulation of the negative regulator p27, are counter balanced by apoptotic checkpoints, such that c-myc over-expression activates the p53 program through the nucleolar tumor suppressor ARF [5, 29, 68, 69]. Deregulation of c-myc has been implicated in the pathogenesis of a number of human cancers and, in different tumor contexts, can occur through gene translocation or amplification, mRNA stabilization, enhanced translation or protein stabilization (reviewed in Dang et al.) [69].

In the case of BL, c-myc deregulation typically results from one of three reciprocal translocations, involving the IgH gene (t(8;14)) in around 80% of cases and the kappa (t(8;22)) or lambda (t(2;8)) IgL genes in the remainder [5, 29, 69]. Where studied, translocations into the light chain loci invariably place the whole c-myc gene some distance from the IgL sequence [5, 29, 52, 69].

In contrast, the anatomy of the t(8:14) translocation falls into one of two broad patterns that tend to correlate with the epidemiologic form of the tumor [5, 17, 29, 52, 69]. Thus, in endemic BL the breakpoint in c-Myc typically occurs more than 100 kb upstream of the first coding exon, and the breakpoint in IgH occurs in the joining region [2, 3, 5, 29, 52, 69].

Again, in sporadic BL and AIDS-BL, the breakpoint in c-Myc often occurs between exons 1 and 2, and the breakpoint in IgH occurs in the switch region [5, 29, 52, 69, 70]. The potential significance of these differences, in terms of the timing of the translocation during B-cell development, has been widely debated, but the issue remains unresolved. [70-72].

Research Efforts and Updates on Myc Gene

There have been several attempts to recapitulate BL in mouse models using Ig-myc fusion transgenes [73-75]. In early work, transgenic mice carrying a wild-type c-myc gene fused to an IgH enhancer developed tumors, but these were of pre-B cell origin and did not resemble classical BL [75]. Notable recent project used a transgene that reconstructed the c-myc/IgL enhancer translocation from a naturally occurring case of BL, where the c-myc gene itself carried mutations [29, 73-75]. This produced mouse B-cell tumors with a histology and cell phenotype closely resembling BL, but which were different in having a naïve (nonmutated) Ig genotype rather than the hypermutated Ig genotype typical of the human tumor [73-75]. These findings with a naturally occurring gene fusion, and earlier reports of c-myc sequence changes in BL, suggest that c-myc gene mutations, arising as a direct result of the translocation itself and/or through inappropriate targeting by the somatic hypermutation machinery that is naturally activated in germinal center cells, render the overexpressed c-myc protein more oncogenic [5, 29, 73-75].

Mechanisms Whereby C-Myc Drives BL Tumorigenesis

The precise mechanisms whereby c-myc drives BL tumorigenesis are still not fully understood. Some insights have come from an *in vitro* reconstruction system in which a lymphoblastoid cell line (LCL), established from normal human B cells using an EBV strain whose transforming function is estrogen-dependent, was transfected with either a constitutive or a tetracycline-regulatable c-myc gene [76-78]. Overexpression of c-myc in these cells renders cell growth independent of EBV and, very interestingly, induces downregulation of LCL-associated cell adhesion and activation molecules and concomitant upregulation of BL-associated germinal center markers such as CD10 and CD38 [79-81].

Such findings reinforce the arguments from transgenic mouse work that c-myc overexpression in B cells can impose a germinal center–like phenotype even though, ironically, normal germinal center cells do not express c-myc [70, 81]; the findings also caution against making the too easy assumption that BL, because it displays a germinal center phenotype, is necessarily of germinal center cell origin. Interestingly, the *in vitro* reconstruction model also showed that c-myc expression imposed on LCL cells a non-immunogenic phenotype typical of BL itself, reducing the expression of HLA molecules and components of the antigen-processing pathway, downregulating many genes involved in the NF-κB response, and impairing the cellular response to type I interferons [77, 80, 81]. This raises the possibility of another role for c-myc in BL pathogenesis, in aiding the tumor's capacity to evade host immune controls [5, 29, 81].

Recent Studies to Determine the Role of C-Myc in Tumorigenesis

More recent studies to determine the role of c-myc in tumorigenesis have used microarray technology to look at the genomic binding sites of c-myc in BL cells. Interestingly, c-myc was found bound to nearly 15% of gene loci tested, consistent with a global role for the protein in determining the malignant BL phenotype [80-82].

Notable among c-myc target genes identified in this study were several involved in driving apoptosis, reflecting the known link between c-myc expression and apoptosis susceptibility seen in normal cells. Indeed, there is evidence both from histologic analysis of tumor biopsies and from tumor explanation in vitro that BL, though a rapidly proliferating tumor, nevertheless also suffers from high rates of apoptosis [5, 29, 80-82].

Matters in Histologic Diagnosis of BL

All forms of BL show a similar histologic appearance, with a malignant population of round monomorphic B cells, interspersed with macrophages that give the tumor histology a "starry sky" pattern (please see Figure 2) [26, 49, 52, 82]. The malignant cells also display an unusually high level of proliferation, indicated by a Ki67 score of greater than 95%, and express combinations of markers (BCL6^{+}, CD10^{+}, CD38^{+}) that are characteristic of germinal center B cells [28, 82], i.e., the stage at which antibody responses mature through somatic hypermutation of immunoglobulin [Ig] genes and Ig class switching. In practice, however, the histologic distinction between classical BL and certain presentations of diffuse large B cell lymphoma (DLBCL) can be difficult to draw [81, 82]. However, distinguishing these pathogenetically distinct entities is important clinically since, compared with DLBCL, the successful treatment of BL requires a much more intensive chemotherapeutic regimen [79-82].

Recent Advances in the Molecular Diagnosis of BL

In light of the above, two recent studies have used microarray technology in an attempt to identify gene expression signatures that distinguish BL, and "Burkitt-like" lymphomas, which have genetic abnormalities and immunophenotype of BL but have atypical morphologic features, from DLBCL [83, 84]. In each study, more than 200 aggressive B-cell lymphomas, previously diagnosed histologically by a panel of expert pathologists, were analysed by gene expression array; in addition, the genetic complexity of these same tumors was assessed either by fluorescent *in situ* hybridization (FISH) analysis to detect c-myc translocations or by array-based comparative genomic hybridization to detect other genetic changes [83, 84]. This expression profiling clearly identified a set of tumors with the molecular signature of BL (mBL); while this signature does indeed overlap with that of normal germinal-center B cells, it is distinct from DLBCL by including high expression of c-myc itself and of a number of c-myc–activated genes [79-84]. Importantly, the molecularly defined mBL tumor set encompassed all those tumors with a classical BL histology, some but not all of the tumors diagnosed as "Burkitt-like," and even a few cases diagnosed as DLBCL by histopathology [79-82, 84].

The powerful combination of gene expression array with genetic analysis made it clear that most cases of molecularly defined BL carried a c-myc/Ig gene translocation, and relatively few if any additional genetic changes detectable by comparative genome hybridization [5, 29, 80-82, 84]. This emphasizes the dominant influence of this translocation on the BL phenotype. Yet interestingly, although high c-myc expression is an integral part of the mBL signature, a few molecularly defined BLs lacked such a translocation, implying that in rare cases the tumor can arise as a result of c-myc deregulation by another route [5, 29, 80-82, 84]. As to the implications of these studies for BL diagnosis, currently it is not practical or cost-efficient to use microarray analysis as a routine diagnostic tool [51, 54, 79-84]. However, the array work has identified additional features of the mBL phenotype, such as TCL1 and BCL6 expression in the absence of CD44 and MUM1, which can be assayed by immunohistochemistry and can augment markers currently in use [82-84].

It is important to note that both of these recent array-based studies were conducted on collections of lymphomas from Western countries and so, by definition, were focusing on sporadic forms of BL. While EBV status was not recorded in the published reports, it is likely that only a minority of the molecularly defined BLs were EBV^+. An important priority for future work will be to determine how closely endemic BL accords to the molecular signature of the sporadic disease and, indeed, whether there are specific changes in cellular gene expression associated with the presence of EBV.

Research in the Treatment Advances of BL

The various research projects in the treatment advances of BL are described and discussed below:

Revelation of New Approaches to Burkitt Lymphoma Treatment and Management

In a study in 2012, by Scientist from the National Cancer Institute (NCI) of the National Institute of Health and undertaken by Staudt and his co-workers uncovered new ways of how BL differs from other lymphomas, and they found different cancer-related genes and pathways that can be targets for future treatments.

The Research Team reported as follows [85]:

- Non-Hodgkin lymphomas are cancers that arise from white blood cells. The disease originates in B cells, which are antibody-producing cells that protect the body against bacteria and viruses. Burkitt lymphoma and diffuse large B-cell lymphoma (DLBCL) are 2 different types of aggressive non-Hodgkin lymphoma that require different treatments.
- The previous work indicated that BL can be readily distinguished from DLBCL based on signatures of gene activity. Notably, the oncogene MYC activates many genes that are more highly expressed in BL than in DLBCL.
- In their study, the team set out to identify genes and pathways that cooperate with *MYC* in BL. They sequenced biopsy samples from 28 patients with sporadic Burkitt lymphoma and 13 different Burkitt lymphoma cell lines. They compared the data to published

data from 80 DLBCL biopsies. They then confirmed their genetic findings through additional sequencing methods and larger sample sizes, results of which were published online in *Nature* on of 12 August 2012.

- The researchers identified some unique genes that were mutated in each disease. The results showed that these lymphomas use fundamentally different mechanisms to become cancerous. It was also noted that for lymphoma patients, TCF3 is needed for B cell function and ID3 is known to inhibit TCF3, and that mutations in these genes were rare in DLBCL.
- Most of the mutations in TCF3 and ID3 led to increased signaling from the B cell receptor, a protein on the B cell surface. These signals promote survival of BL tumor cells by turning on one of the most frequently activated signaling pathways in human cancer, the PI(3) kinase pathway.
- It was further noted that development of PI(3) kinase inhibitors for use in cancer patients is well underway, but no inhibitor has yet been tested in patients with BL.

Less Toxic Alternative to Standard Treatment for Adults with BL

On 26 May 2020, it was reported that researchers at the NCI, part of NIH have identified an alternative treatment regimen that is less toxic than standard dose-intensive chemotherapy, which is found to be highly effective for adults with BL across all age groups and independent of HIV status. In addition to being better tolerated, the regimen, called dose-adjusted (DA) EPOCH-R, is already an option for diffuse large B-cell lymphomas and can be administered in an outpatient setting. The report also stated as follows [86]:

- The study was conducted at 22 research centers across the USA. It was noted that The DA-EPOCH-R regimen was originally developed by NCI researchers led by "Wyndham Wilson, M.D., at the NIH Clinical Center in Bethesda, Maryland," USA.

- The research team pointed out that they know that BL "is curable with dose-intensive chemotherapy, but that treatment can be acutely toxic for adult patients." The research team asserted that with this current findings that they "not only have a potentially curative treatment option for these patients that is less toxic, but one that appears effective for most adults, including elderly patients and those with HIV and other comorbidities who might not be able to receive standard treatment."
- It was again emphasised that BL is a rare but aggressive B-cell lymphoma that is more common in children than adults. The dose-intensive chemotherapy that's been developed to cure BL in pediatric patients is much better tolerated by children than adults, who can have severe side effects, especially if they are older or have other serious health conditions, such as being infected with HIV. It is generally noted that people living with HIV/AIDS have an increased risk for BL.
- In addition, NCI researchers have tested several approaches to determine whether less toxic treatments could still be effective for Burkitt lymphoma in adults. It was reported that in an earlier pilot study with 30 adult patients treated only at NCI, the DA-EPOCH-R chemotherapy regimen was effective. The DA-EPOCH-R regimen was tailored to an individual patient's ability to tolerate chemotherapy. The regimen infuses chemotherapy over 96 hours for each cycle, and "dose-adjusted" means that later cycles can use higher doses of chemotherapy if it is well tolerated. This is compared to "dose-intensive" chemotherapy, which uses very high doses in all patients from the beginning.
- It was stated that the researchers conducted a larger, multicenter phase two study, enrolling 113 patients identified as having low- or high-risk disease, based on characteristics such as tumor bulk and performance status in order to confirm their findings. The median age of the participants was 49 years, and 62% were 40 years or older.

- At a median follow-up of almost five years, the researchers calculated that the four-year rate of event-free survival was 84.5%, meaning that percentage of patients had not seen any sign of their cancer's return. Overall survival was 87%. For low-risk patients, event-free survival was 100%, and for high-risk patients it was 82%.
- The treatment was effective across age groups, including patients in their 70s and 80s, and regardless of HIV status. The treatment was well-tolerated with a relatively low number of patients experiencing the severe side effects commonly associated with dose-intensive chemotherapy.
- These finding suggest that highly dose-intensive chemotherapy may not be necessary for cute, and that carefully defined low-risk patients may be treated with limited chemotherapy. Furthermore, patients can receive EPOCH-R in an outpatient setting, an alternative to the prolonged hospitalization required to receive dose-intensive chemotherapy.
- It was further reported that five treatment-related deaths occurred in the study. The researchers found that patients in the study who had disease in the central nervous system, specifically in cerebrospinal fluid (CSF), had the highest risk of treatment-related death or treatment failure. As a result, the researcher's contended that further studies are warranted to determine how best to treat patients with CSF involvement.

Discussion

In this chapter, we have evaluated the etiology, classification, pathologic issues, diagnosis, clinical manifestations, epidemiology, prognosis, and treatment issues of BL, including exploring research efforts in the diagnosis and treatments of the disease, using clinical systematic review research method, and the analysis of experts' opinions. We found that BL is a highly aggressive, but potentially curable type of B-cell NHL with a cellular doubling time of 24-48 hours. This is similar to the findings of Ally et al., in 2019 [87].

It was also noted that BL, which was first described by Denis Burkitt as an obscure tumor of African children [3, 87], has since taken a special position as the first human tumor whose pathogenesis could be linked both to an oncogenic virus, EBV, and to the activation of a specific cellular oncogene, c-myc [4, 5, 15-17, 19, 29, 33-39, 40-43, 69, 73, 78, 79, 82, 87]. Scientists and clinicians continue to be intrigued on how these factors complement one another in the oncogenic process, and what other factors play a role in the pathogenesis of BL [79, 82, 87].

Derived from B-cell germinal centers [88], BL was first described as a distinct clinical entity in 1958 [3, 87, 88]. It was one of the first human tumors found to have a relationship with a viral infection, EBV [2, 3, 39, 43, 82, 87, 88]. BL is also associated with a chromosomal translocation that activates the MYC protooncogene and is the first lymphoma reported to be associated with Human 1 mmunodeficiencv Virus (HIV) infection [89]. BL is one of the most common pediatric malignancies in sub-Saharan African countries, with an incidence rate as high as 4.7 cases per year for males and 3.0 cases per year for females (per 100, 000 children under 15 years of age) [90]. Three subtypes of BL are recognized: Endemic, Sporadic, and Immunodeficiency associated [2, 3, 11-13, 53, 90].

Endemic (African) BL, which mainly occurs in equatorial Africa (it also occurs in Papua Guinea), is the most common subtype in childhood and boys are more likely to be affected than girls (approximate ratio of 2:1) [3, 6, 21, 22, 54, 59, 61, 89, 90]. Endemic BL accounts for nearly 30%-50% of all childhood cases [3, 91, 92], and infection by EBV is found in nearly 100% of all patients with endemic BL [93]. Moreover, although Plasmodium falciparum is not an agent of the MYC proto-oncogene, its possible oncogenic development of BL has been demonstrated through the shared geographic distribution of BL and malaria [94].

Sporadic BL is primarily observed in young adults, with an incidence of 1%-2% of all lymphomas occurring at a median age of 30 (M:F is 3:1 or 4:1), although in pediatrics, it represents 40% of all lymphomas [6, 3, 21, 22, 54, 59, 61, 89, 94]. Moreover, EBV is detectable in <30% of sporadic

BL [95-97] and the disease is more common in Caucasians than Africans or Asian-Americans. It may also be common in some areas of Central America (Guatemala) [98].

Immunodeficiency-associated BL, the third subtype, is seen primarily in HIV patients, often occurring as the initial clinical manifestation of AIDS. Indeed, an EBV infection is detected in approximately 40% of cases. Interestingly, immunodeficiencyassociated BL is unlike other HIV-associated B-cell lymphomas because it typically occurs in patients with CD4 counts greater than 200 cells, per pL. As a result of antiretroviral therapy, the incidence has decreased, but it may also be seen in other immunodeficiency states (for example, post organ transplant). These patients typically present with BL 4-5 years after organ transplantation [98, 99].

In addition, two seminal observations underpin the status of BL as a key model for the understanding of multistage tumorigenesis [3, 28, 69, 100]:

- The discovery in the 1960s of BL association with EBV became a foundation stone of human tumor virology and has presaged four decades of research in which the full oncogenic potential of this virus has slowly been realised.
- The discovery in the 1980s of c-myc/Ig gene fusions at the site of t(8:14), t(2:8) and t(8:22) translocations in BL united the worlds of cyto- and molecular genetics, setting a path that would open up the molecular basis of oncogenic change in many other tumor contexts.

Ironically, so wide became the vistas in both the above fields as to divert attention away from BL itself. The present study indicates how, more recently, that focus has been restored in a way that again emphasizes the continued potential of BL to reveal new insights [3, 28, 69, 100]. Hence, the examination in transgenic mouse models of c-myc–driven B-cell lymphomagenesis in the research into the advances in diagnosis and treatment of BL section in this article is identifying key aspects of c-myc function that are relevant to BL pathogenesis, with a focus on the decoupling of c-myc's proproliferative and pro-apoptotic effects [5, 29, 69, 73, 78, 79, 82, 100].

Similarly, projects in the EBV field are now revealing the capacity of non–growth-transforming forms of EBV latency to confer protection from apoptosis [4, 15, 16, 19, 33-39, 40-43, 79, 82, 100]. While not yet fully understood at a mechanistic level, these findings clearly point to ways in which EBV's contribution to BL pathogenesis might be reconciled with the primacy of c-myc as the driver of tumor growth [29, 69, 73, 78, 79, 82, 100].

Despite these advances, it is clear that many questions still remain to be resolved. These include questions about [3, 17, 28, 69, 100]:

- the timing of EBV's contribution vis-à-vis that of the c-myc translocation
- the influence of EBV on the molecular signature of the tumor
- the identity of the BL progenitor cell and whether its germinal center–like phenotype truly reflects the tumor's origin
- the mechanisms by which malaria and HIV increase BL risk

Addressing these issues will require the concerted efforts of many disciplines, the intelligent use of both *in vivo* and *in vitro* models, and a renewed focus on the analysis of primary tumor material from endemic, sporadic and AIDS-associated forms of the disease.

Our work differs from the work of other groups because we believe that we are the first team to look into the diagnosis, treatment, epidemiology, prognosis, including trends and issues in research and innovations, and healthcare issues in BL in details. Generally, we observed that BL is fatal if left untreated. In children, prompt intensive chemotherapy usually cures BL, leading to long-term survival rates of 60% to 90%. In adult patients, results are more variable [59, 61, 89, 100]. Overall, prompt treatment is associated with long-term survival rates of 70% to 80% [88, 100]. Our analysis of the research efforts into the diagnosis and treatment approaches in BL showed that progress has been made in advancement of techniques for better outcomes of patient care and management, and there are more investigations needed in order to improve the prognosis of BL for patients and their families [20, 55, 58, 59, 61, 88, 89, 100].

There is a limitation in our current review in that if we would have had more time, we would have explored further on the areas of all advances in the diagnosis and treatments of BL starting back from the historical times to current period in order to compare the efficiency and effectiveness of each approach, which would add towards the creation of evidence-based guidelines for the diagnosis and treatment/management of BL in the changing World. So this would be the subject of our future work.

Conclusion

BL is a cancer of the lymphatic system, particularly B lymphocytes found in the germinal center. It is named after Denis Parsons Burkitt, the British/Irish surgeon who first described the disease in 1958 while working in equatorial Africa. Thus BL is a rare but highly aggressive (fast-growing) B-cell non-Hodgkin lymphoma (NHL). This disease may affect the jaw, central nervous system, bowel, kidneys, ovaries, or other organs. BL may spread to the central nervous system (CNS). Translocation (a type of rearrangement) of a gene called MYC is a hallmark of BL, making this an important finding for diagnosis. In adults, BL is often indistinguishable from diffuse large B-cell lymphoma (DLBCL)-another aggressive B-cell lymphoma. Accurate diagnosis of BL is critical because BL and DLBCL are treated differently. That is why it is strongly recommended that both clinicians and patients seek an opinion from an expert in lymphoma. Localized tumours respond well to chemotherapy; long-term disease-free survival rates are about 90 percent for patients with less- advanced disease (stages I or II) and 80 to 90 percent for patients with more-advanced disease (stages III and IV). Involvement of the central nervous system, however, can lead to a far more serious prognosis. The overall cure rate for BL in developed countries is about 90%, but worse in low-income countries. BL is uncommon in adults, in whom it has a worse prognosis. Future work will involve exploring current advances in the treatments of BL and trends and issues in this area of cancer.

REFERENCES

[1] Kingsley-Godwin D.E.C.C.O.H. and Kingsley-Godwin M. J. (2013). Burkitt's Lymphoma: Examination of Aetiology, Pathophysiology, Histopathology, Treatment and Health Issues. *The North and West London Journal of General Practice* 10(2): 24 - 32,

[2] Molyneux E. M., Rochford R., Griffin B., Newton R., Jackson G., Menon G., Harrison C. J., Israels T. (2012), Bailey S. Burkitt's lymphoma. *Lancet* 379 (9822): 1234-44.

[3] Burkitt D. (1958). "A sarcoma involving the jaws in African children." *The British Journal of Surgery* 46 (197): 218-23.

[4] Dojcinov, S. D., Fend, F., Quintanilla-Martinez, L. (7 March 2018). "EBV-Positive Lymphoproliferations of B- T- and NK-Cell Derivation in Non-Immunocompromised Hosts." *Pathogens* (Basel, Switzerland) 7 (1): 28.

[5] Haberl S., Haferlach T., Stengel A., Jeromin S., Kern W., Haferlach C. (2016). MYC rearranged B-cell neoplasms: Impact of genetics on classification. *Cancer Genet*. 209 (10):431-439.

[6] Grande B. M., Gerhard D. S., Jiang A., Griner N. B., Abramson J. S., Alexander T. B., Allen H., Ayers L. W., Bethony J. M., Bhatia K., Bowen J., Casper C., Choi J. K., Culibrk L., Davidsen T. M., Dyer M. A., Gastier-Foster J. M., Gesuwan P., Greiner T. C., Gross T. G., Hanf B., Harris N. L., He Y., Irvin J. D., Jaffe E. S., Jones S. J. M., Kerchan P., Knoetze N., Leal F. E., Lichtenberg T. M., Ma Y., Martin J. P., Martin M. R., Mbulaiteye S. M., Mullighan C. G., Mungall A. J., Namirembe C., Novik K., Noy A., Ogwang M. D., Omoding A., Orem J., Reynolds S. J., Rushton C. K., Sandlund J. T., Schmitz R., Taylor C., Wilson W. H., Wright G. W., Zhao E. Y., Marra M. A., Morin R. D., Staudt L. M. (2019). Genome-wide

discovery of somatic coding and noncoding mutations in pediatric endemic and sporadic Burkitt lymphoma. *Blood* 133 (12):1313-132.

[7] Sandlund J. T. (2012). Burkitt lymphoma: staging and response evaluation. *Br J Haematol.* 156 (6):761-5.

[8] Marjerrison S., Fernandez C. V., Price V. E., Njume E., Hesseling P. (2012). The use of ultrasound in endemic Burkitt lymphoma in Cameroon. *Pediatr Blood Cancer* 58 (3):352-5.

[9] Vandenbroucke J. P., von Elm E., Altman D. G., Gotzsche P. C., Mulrow C. D., Pocock S. J., Poole C., Schlesselman J. J., Egger M., Initiative S. (2014). Strengthening the reporting of observational studies in epidemiology (STROBE): explanation and elaboration. *Int J Surg.* 12:1500-1524. doi:10.10l6/j.ijsu.2014.07.014.

[10] Higgins J. P., Thompson S. G., Deeks J. J., Altman D. G. (2003). Measuring inconsistency in meta-analyses. *BMJ*; 327: 557-560. doi:10.1136/bmj.327.7414.557.

[11] *Burkitt lymphoma.* https://www.msdmanuals.com/professional/hematology-and-oncology/lymphomas/burkitt-lymphoma Accessed on April 17 2021.

[12] Brady G., MacArthur G. J., Farrell P. J. (December 2007). "Epstein-Barr virus and Burkitt lymphoma." *Journal of Clinical Pathology.* 60 (12): 1397-1402.

[13] Bellan C., Lazzi S., De Falco G., Nyongo A., Giordano A., Leoncini L. (March 2003). "Burkitt's lymphoma: new insights into molecular pathogenesis." *J Clin. Pathol.* 56 (3): 188-92.

[14] Casulo C., Friedberg J. (September 2015). "Treating Burkitt Lymphoma in Adults." *Current Hematologic Malignancy Reports.* 10 (3): 266-71.

[15] Vockerodt M., Yap L. F., Shannon-Lowe C., Curley H., Wei W., Vrzalikova K., Murray P. G. (January 2015). "The Epstein-Barr virus and the pathogenesis of lymphoma." *The Journal of Pathology.* 235 (2): 312-22.

[16] Navari M., Etebari M., De Falco G., Ambrosio M. R., Gibellini D., Leoncmi L., Piccaluga P. P. (2015) "The presence of Epstein-Barr virus significantly impacts the transcriptional profile in

immunodeficienc-associated bukitt lymphoma." *Frontiers in Microbiology* 6:556.

[17] Rezk S. A., Zhao X., Weiss L. M., (September 2018). "Epstein-Barr virus (EBV)-associated lymphoid proliferations, a 2018 update." *Human Pathology* 79:18-41. doi:10.1016/ij.humpath.2018.05.020. PMID 29885408.

[18] Turgeon M. L., "Clinical hematology: theory and procedures." In *Frequency of lymphoid neoplasms.* (Source: Modified from WHO Blue Book on Tumour of Hematopoietic and Lymphoid Tissues. 2001, p. 2001). Hagerstown, MD: Lippincott Williams & Wilkins, 2005: 283. ISBN 0-7817-5007-5.

[19] Pannone G., Zamparese R., Pace M., Pedicillo, Maria C., Simona S., Pasquale E. M., Donofrio V., Franco R., De Chiara A., Aquino G., Bucci P., Bucci E., Santoro A., Bufo P., (2014). "The role of EBV in the pathogenesis of Burkitt's Lvmphoma: an Italian hospital based survey." *Infectious Agents and Cancer* 9 (1): 34. doi:l0.1186/1750-9378- 9-34. ISSN: 1750-9378. PMC 4216353. PMID 25364378.

[20] Linch D. C. (2012) Burkitt lymphoma in adults. *Br J Haematol.* 156(6):693-703.

[21] Dozzo M., Carobolante F., Donisi P. M., Scattolin A., Maino E., Sancetta R., Viero P., Bassan R.. (2017). Burkitt lymphoma in adolescents and young adults: management challenges. *Adolesc Health Med Ther.* 8: 11-29.

[22] Kelly G. L., Rickinson A. L. (2007) Burkitt Lymphoma: Revisiting the Pathogenesis of a Virus-Associated Malignancy. Pediatric Hematologic Malignancies: Non-Hodgkin Lymphoma| January 1, 2007. *Hematology Am Soc Hematol Educ Program* 2007 (1): 277–284. https://doi.org/10.1182/asheducation-2007.1.277.

[23] Haberl S., Haferlach T., Stengel A., Jeromin S., Kern W., Haferlach C., (2016) MYC rearranged B-cell neoplasms: Impact of genetics on classification. *Cancer Genet.* 209 (10):431-439.

[24] Hoffman R. 2009. *Hematology: basic principles and practice* (PDF) (5th ed.). Philadelphia, PA: Churchill Livingstone/Elsevier. (Hoffman 2009, 1304-1305). ISBN 978-0-443- 06715-0.

[25] Liu D., Shimonov J, Primanneni S., Lai Y., Ahmed T., Seiter K. (2007). "t(8:14:18): a 3-wav chromosome translocation in two patients with Burkitt's lvmphoma/leukemia." *Mol. Cancer* 6 (1): 35. doi:10.1186/1476-4598-6-35. PMC 1904237. PMID 17547754.

[26] Smardova J., Grochova D., Fabian P., et al. (October 2008). "An unusual p53 mutation detected in Burkitt's lvmphoma: 30 bp duplication." *Oncol. Rep.* 20 (4): 773-8. doi:10.3892/ or 00000073. PMID 18813817.

[27] Tierney R., Nagra J., Hutchings I., et al. (2007). Epstein-Barr virus exploits Bsap/Pax5 to achieve the B cell specificity of its growth-transforming programme. *J Virol.*; 81:10092–10100.

[28] Rickinson A. B., Kieff E. "Epstein-Barr virus." In *Fields Virology. Vol. II (5th ed.)*. edited by D. M. Knipe and P. M. Howley, 2655–2700. Philadelphia: Lippincott, Williams & Wilkins, 2007.

[29] Pajic A., Staege M. S., Dudziak D., et al. (2001). Antagonistic effects of c-myc and Epstein-Barr virus latent genes on the phenotype of human B cells. *Int J Cancer* 93:810–816.

[30] Kelly G., Bell A., Rickinson A. (2002). Epstein-Barr virus-associated Burkitt lymphomagenesis selects for downregulation of the nuclear antigen EBNA2. *Nat Med.*8:1098–1104.

[31] Kelly G. L., Milner A. E., Baldwin G. S., Bell A. I., Rickinson A. B., (2006). Three restricted forms of Epstein-Barr virus latency counteracting apoptosis in c-myc-expressing Burkitt lymphoma cells. *Proc Natl Acad Sci USA* 103:14935–14940.

[32] Shimizu N., Tanabe-Tochikura A., Kuroiwa Y., Takada K. (1994). Isolation of Epstein-Barr virus (EBV)-negative cell clones from the EBV-positive Burkitt's lymphoma (BL) line Akata: malignant phenotypes of BL cells are dependent on EBV. *J Virol.* 68:6069–6073.

[33] Ruf I. K., Rhyne P. W., Yang H., et al. (1999). Epstein-barr virus regulates c-MYC, apoptosis, and tumorigenicity in Burkitt lymphoma. *Mol Cell Biol.* 19:1651–1660.

[34] Kennedy G., Komano J., Sugden B. (2003). Epstein-Barr virus provides a survival factor to Burkitt's lymphomas. *Proc Natl Acad Sci U S A*. 100:14269.

[35] Komano J., Maruo. S, Kurozumi K., Oda T., Takada K. (1999). Oncogenic role of Epstein-Barr virus-encoded RNAs in Burkitt's lymphoma cell line *Akata. J Virol.* 73:9827–9831.

[36] Komano J., Sugiura M., Takada K. (1998). Epstein-Barr virus contributes to the malignant phenotype and to apoptosis resistance in Burkitt's lymphoma cell line *Akata. J Virol.* 72:9150–9156.

[37] Ruf I. K., Rhyne P. W., Yang C., Cleveland J. L., Sample J. T. (2000). Epstein-Barr virus small RNAs potentiate tumorigenicity of Burkitt lymphoma cells independently of an effect on apoptosis. *J Virol.* 74:10223–10228.

[38] Kelly G. L., Milner A. E., Tierney R. J., et al. (2005). Epstein-Barr virus nuclear antigen 2 (EBNA2) gene deletion is consistently linked with EBNA3A, -3B, and -3C expression in Burkitt's lymphoma cells and with increased resistance to apoptosis. *J Virol.* 79:10709–10717.

[39] Leao M., Anderton E., Wade M., Meekings K., Allday M. J. (2007). Epstein-barr virus-induced resistance to drugs that activate the mitotic spindle assembly checkpoint in Burkitt's lymphoma cells. *J Virol*. 81:248–260.

[40] Ioachim H. L., Cronin W., Roy M., Maya M., (1990). Persistent lymphadenopathies in people at high risk for HIV infection—clinicopathological correlations and long-term follow-up in 79 cases. *Am J Clin Pathol*. 93:208.

[41] Piriou E. R., van Dort K., Nanlohy N. M., Miedema F., van Oers M. H., van Baarle D. (2004). Altered EBV viral load setpoint after HIV seroconversion is in accordance with lack of predictive value of EBV load for the occurrence of AIDS-related non-Hodgkin lymphoma. *J Immunol.* 172:6931–6937.

[42] Moormann A. M., Chelimo K., Sumba O. P., et al. (2005). Exposure to holoendemic malaria results in elevated Epstein-Barr virus loads in children. *J Infect Dis*. 191:1233–1238.

[43] Donati D., Espmark E., Kironde F., et al. (2006). Clearance of circulating Epstein-Barr virus DNA in children with acute malaria after antimalaria treatment. *J Infect Dis.* 193:971–977.

[44] Rochford R., Cannon M. J., Moormann A. M. (2005). Endemic Burkitt's lymphoma: a polymicrobial disease? *Nat Rev Microbiol.* 3:182–187.

[45] Moormann A. M., Chelimo K., Sumba P. O., Tisch D. J., Rochford R., Kazura J. W. (2007). Exposure to holoendemic malaria results in suppression of Epstein-Barr virus-specific T cell immunosurveillance in Kenyan children. *J Infect Dis*. 195:799–808.

[46] Donati D., Zhang L. P., Chene A., et al. (2004). Identification of a polyclonal B-cell activator in Plasmodium falciparum. *Infect Immun.*72:5412–5418.

[47] Donati D., Mok B., Chene A., et al. (2006). Increased B cell survival and preferential activation of the memory compartment by a malaria polyclonal B cell activator. *J Immunol.*77:3035–3044.

[48] Chene A., Donati D., Guerreiro-Cacais A. O., et al. A molecular link between malaria and Epstein-Barr virus reactivation. *PLoS Pathog.*3:e80.

[49] *Burkitt lymphoma.* https://www.researchgate.net/figure/The-Starrv-skv-pattem-of-Burkitts-lvmphoma-The-tumour-cells-of-B-lvmphoblasts-which fig1 263292845 Accessed on April 12 2021.

[50] *Burkitt lymphoma.* https://basicmedicalkev.com/burkitt-lvmphoma-2/ Accessed on April 12 2021.

[51] Bellan C., Lazzi S., De Falco G., Nyongo A., Giordano A., Leoncini L (March 2003). "Burkitt's lymphoma: new insights into molecular pathogenesis." *J. Clin. Pathol.* 56 (3): 188–92. doi:10.1136/jcp.56. 3.188. PMC 1769902. PMID 12610094.

[52] Fujita S., Buziba N., Kumatori A., Senba M., Yamaguchi A. Toriyama K. (mAy 2004). "Early_stage of Epstein-Barr virus lytic infection leading to the "starry sky" pattern formation in endemic Burkitt's lytnnhoma" *Arch. Pathol. Lab Med.* 128(5): 549-52.doi:10543-216Sf2004) 128<549: SOEVL >2.0CO;2(interactive 2021-01-18).PMID 15086279.

[53] Steven H. Swerdlow. *WHO classification of tumours of haematopoietic and lymphoid tissues.* World Health Organization classification of tumours. Lyon, France: International Agency for Research on Cancer, 2008. ISBN 978-92-832-2431-0.

[54] Naresh K. N., et al. (2011). *Lymphomas in sub-Saharan Africa – what can we learn and how can we help in improving diagnosis, managing patients and fostering translational research?* doi:10.1111/j.1365-2141.2011.08772.x. Accessed on April 12 2021.

[55] Thomas D. A., Faderl S., O'Brien S., Bueso-Ramos C., Cortes J., Garcia-Manero G., Giles F. J., Verstovsek S., Wierda W. G., Pierce S.A., Shan J., Brandt M., Hagemeister F. B., Keating M. l., Cabanillas F., Kantaijian H. (2006). Chemoimmunotherapy with hyper-CVAD plus rituximab for the treatment of adult Burkitt and Burkitt-type lymphoma or acute lymphoblastic leukemia. *Cancer* 106 (7): 1569-80.

[56] Mead G. M., Sydes M. R., Walewski J, Grigg A., Hatton C. S., Pescosta N., Guarnaccia C., Lewis M. S., McKendrick J., Stenning S. P., Wright D., Norbert P., UKLG LY06 collaborators. (2002). An international evaluation of CODOX-M and CODOX-M alternating with IVAC in adult Burkitt's lymphoma: results of United Kingdom Lymphoma Group LY06 study. *Ann Oncol.* 13 (8): 1264-74.

[57] Barnes J. A., Lacasce A. S., Feng Y., Toomey C. E., Neuberg D., Michaelson J. S., Hochberg E. P., Abramson J. S. (2011). Evaluation of the addition of rituximab to CODOX-M/IVAC for Burkitt's lymphoma: a retrospective analysis. *Ann Oncol.* 22 (8): 1859-64.

[58] Dunleavy K., Pittaluga S., Shovlin M., Steinberg S. M., Cole D., Grant C., Widemann B., Staudt L. M., Jaffe E. S., Little R. F., Wilson W. H.. Low-intensity therapy in adults with Burkitt's lymphoma. *N Engl J Med.* 369 (20): 1915-25.

[59] Gross T. G., Hale G. A., He W., Camitta B. M., Sanders J. E., Cairo M. S., Hayashi R. J., Termuhlen A. M., Zhang M. J., Davies S. M., Eapen M. (2010). Hematopoietic stem cell transplantation for refractory or recurrent non-Hodgkin lymphoma in children and adolescents. *Biol Blood Marrow Transplant.* 16(2):223-30.

[60] Barnes J. A., LaCasce A. S., Feng Y. et al. (2011), Evaluation of the addition of rituximab to CODOX-M/ IVAC for Burkitt's lymphoma: a retrospective analysis. *Annals of Oncology.* 22 (8): 1859-64. doi'JO. 1093/annnnc/mdq677. PMID 21339382.

[61] Rodney R., Arnold S., Cairo M. S. (2012). Risk factorand treatment of chldood and adolescent Burkitt lymphoma/leukaemia." *British Journal of Haematology* 156 (6): 730-743. doi:10.111/j.1365-2141.2011.09024.x. PMID 22260323. S2CID 6418151.

[62] *Burkitt Lvmphoma and Burkittdike Lvmphoma: Practice Essentials, Background, Etiology and Pathophysiology* 29 June 2017. Accessed April 12 2021 - via eMedicine.

[63] *Burkitt Lymphoma.* http://www.bhs.be/frontend/fi1es/userfiles/files/Guidelmes/Burkitts_Lymphoma_2015.pdf. Accessed on April 12 2021.

[64] Wilson W. H., Kieron Dunleavy K., Pittaluga S., Hegde U., Grant N., Seth M. Steinberg S. M., Raffeld M., Gutierrez M., Chabner B. A., Staudt L., Jaffe E. S., Janik J. E. (2008). Phase II Study of Dose-Adiusted EPOCH-Rituximab in Untreated Diffuse Large B-cell Lvmphoma with Analysis of Germinal Center and Post-Germinal Center Biomarkers. *Journal of Clinical Oncology* 26(16):2717-2724. doi:10.1200/JCO.2007.13.1391. PMC 2409217. PMID 18378569.

[65] Yustein J. T., Dang C. V. (2007). Biology and treatment of Burkitfs lymphoma. *Curr. Opin. Hematol.* 14 (4): 375-81.doi:10.1097/MOH ObOl3e3281bccdee. PMID 17534164. S2CID 8778208.

[66] Shiramizu B., Goldman S., Smith L., Agsalda-Garcia M., Galardy P., Perkins S. L., Frazer Ж., Sanger W., Anderson J. R., Gross T. G., Weinstein H., Harrison L., Barth M. J., Mussolin L., Cairo M. S.. (2015). Impact of persistent minimal residual disease post-consolidation therapy in children and adolescents with advanced Burkitt leukaemia: a Children's Oncology Group Pilot Study Report. *Br J Haematol.* 170 (3):367-71.

[67] *NIH study shows Burkitt lvmphoma is molecularlv distinct from other lymphomas*. National Cancer Institute. Archived from the original on 2012-08-16. Accessed on April 12 2021.

[68] Staudt L. et al. (2012). Burkitt Lvmphoma Pathogenesis and Therapeutic Targets from Structural and Functional Genomics. *Nature* 490 (7418): 116-120. Bibcode: 2012Natur.490. 116S. doi:10.1038/nature11378. PMC 3609867. PMID 22885699.

[69] Dang C. V., O'Donnell K. A., Zeller K. I., Nguyen T., Osthus R. C., Li F. (2006). The c-Myc target gene network. *Semin Cancer Biol.* 16:253–264.

[70] Magrath I. (1990). The pathogenesis of Burkitt's lymphoma. *Adv Cancer Res*. 55:133–270.

[71] Klein U., Tu Y., Stolovitzky G. A. et al. (2003). Transcriptional analysis of the B cell germinal center reaction. *Proc Natl Acad Sci U S A*. 100: 2639–2644.

[72] Goossens T., Klein U., Kuppers R. (1998). Frequent occurrence of deletions and duplications during somatic hypermutation: implications for oncogene translocations and heavy chain disease. *Proc Natl Acad Sc USA*. 5:2463–2468.

[73] Adams J. M., Harris A. W., Pinkert C. A. et al. (1985). The c-myc oncogene driven by immunoglobulin enhancers induces lymphoid malignancy in transgenic mice. *Nature*. 318:533–538.

[74] Kovalchuk A. L., Qi C. F., Torrey T. A. et al. (2000). Burkitt lymphoma in the mouse. *J Exper Med.* 192:1183–1190.

[75] Zhu D., Qi C. F., Morse H. C. 3rd, Janz S., Stevenson F. K. (2005). Deregulated expression of the Myc cellular oncogene drives development of mouse "Burkitt-like" lymphomas from naive B cells. *Blood* 105:2135–2137.

[76] Pajic A., Spitkovsky D., Christoph B. et al. (2000). Cell cycle activation by c-myc in a burkitt lymphoma model cell line. *Int J Cancer* 87:787–793.

[77] Polack A., Hortnagel K., Pajic A. et al. (1996). C-myc activation renders proliferation of Epstein-Barr virus (EBV)-transformed cells independent of EBV nuclear antigen 2 and latent membrane protein 1. *Proc Natl Acad Sci USA*. 93:10411–10416.

[78] Schuhmacher M., Staege M. S., Pajic A. et al. (1999). Control of cell growth by c-Myc in the absence of cell division. *Curr Biol.* 9:1255–1258.

[79] Pajic A., Staege M. S., Dudziak D. et al. (2001). Antagonistic effects of c-myc and Epstein-Barr virus latent genes on the phenotype of human B cells. *Int J Cancer* 93:810–816.

[80] Schlee M., Holzel M., Bernard S. et al. (2007). C-myc activation impairs the NF-kappaB and the interferon response: implications for the pathogenesis of Burkitt's lymphoma. *Int J Cancer* 120:1387–1395.

[81] Staege M. S., Lee S. P., Frisan T. et al. (2002). MYC overexpression imposes a nonimmunogenic phenotype on Epstein-Barr virus-infected B cells. *Proc Natl Acad Sci USA.* 99:4550–4555.

[82] Li Z., Van Calcar S., Qu C., Cavenee W. K., Zhang M. Q., Ren B. (2003). A global transcriptional regulatory role for c-Myc in Burkitt's lymphoma cells. *Proc Natl Acad Sci USA.* 100:8164–8169.

[83] Dave S. S., Fu K., Wright G. W. et al. (2006). Molecular diagnosis of Burkitt's lymphoma. *N Engl J Med.* 354:2431–2442.

[84] Hummel M., Bentink S., Berger H. et al. (2006). A biologic definition of Burkitt's lymphoma from transcriptional and genomic profiling. *N Engl J Med.* 354:2419–2430.

[85] *New Approaches in Burkitt Lymphoma* from: https://www.nih.gov/news-events/nih-research-matters/study-suggests-new-approaches-burkitt-lymphoma Published on September 17, 2012. Accessed on April 17 2021.

[86] *Study confirms effective-less toxic alternative standard treatment for adult Burkitt Lymphoma* from: https://www.nih.gov/news-events/news-releases/study-confirms-effective-less-toxic-alternative-standard-treatment-adults-burkitt-lymphoma Accessed on April 17 2021.

[87] Ally et al. (2019). Treatment Advances for Burkitt Lymphoma. Published in *Open Access Journal of Leukemia* 7(1) published at: https://www.longdom.org/open-access/treatment-advances-for-burkitt-lvmphoma.pdf. Accessed on April 12 2021.

[88] Jacobson C., Lacasce A. (2018). How I treat Burkitt lymphoma in adults. *Blood* 124 (19): 2913-2921.

[89] O'Conor G. T., Davies J. N. (1960). Malignant tumors in African children. With special reference to malignant lymphoma. *J Pediatr.* 56: 526-535.

[90] Orem J., Mbidde E. K., Lambert B., Sanjose S., Weiderpass E. (2007). Burkitt's lymphoma in Africa, a review of the epidemiology and etiology. *Afr Health Sci.* 7 (3): 166-175.

[91] Magrath I. (2012). Epidemiology: Clues to the pathogenesis of Burkitt lymphoma. *Br J Haematol.* 156 (6): 744-756.

[92] Ogwang M. D., Bhatia K., Bigger R. J., Mbulaiteye S. M. (2008). Incidence and geographic distribution of endemic Burkitt lymphoma in northern Uganda revisited *Int J Cancer* 123(11):2658-2663.

[93] de-The G., Geser A., Day N. E., Tukei P. M., Williams E. H., Beri D.P. et al. (1978). Epidemiological evidence for causal relationship between Epstein-Barr virus and Burkitt's lymphoma from Ugandan prospective study. *Nature* 274 (5673):756-761.

[94] Geser A., Brubaker G., Draper C. C. (1989). Effect of a malaria suppression program on the incidence of African Burkitt's lymphoma. *Am J Epidemiol.* 129 (4):740-752.

[95] Morton L. M., Wang S. S., Devesa S. S., Hartge P., Weisenburger D. D., Linet M. S. (2006). Lymphoma incidence patterns by WHO subtype in the United States, 1992-2001. *Blood.* 107 (l):265-276.

[96] Smith A., Howell D., Patmore R., Jack A., Roman E. (2011). Incidence of haematological malignancy by sub-type: A report from the Haematological Malignancy Research Network. *Br J Cancer* 105 (11): 1684-1692.

[97] Hanson S. (2010). Gender and mobility: new approaches for informing sustainability. *Gend Place Cult.* 17:5-23.

[98] Laurini J. A., Perry A. M., Boilesen E., Diebold J., MacLennan K.A., Muller-Hermelink H. K. et al. (2012). Classification of non-Hodgkin lymphoma in Central and South America: A review of 1028 cases. *Blood.* 120 (24):4795-4801.

[99] Shiels M. S., Pfeiffer R. M., Hall H. I., Li J., Morton L. M., Goedert J. J. et al. (2011). Proportions of Kaposi sarcoma, selected non-Hodgkin lymphomas, and cervical cancer in the United States occurring in persons with AIDS, 1980-2007. *JAMA.* 305.1450-1459.

[100] https://ashpublications.org/hematology/article/2007/1/277/19208/Burkitt-Lymphoma-Revisiting-the-Pathogenesis-of-a Accessed on April 17 April.

BIOGRAPHICAL SKETCHES

Daniella E.C.C.O.H. Kingsley-Godwin

Affiliation (s):

- London Medical Academy, London, England, United Kingdom
- Association of health Care Professionals and the International Association of Health Care Professionals (IAHCP) Society, London, England, United Kingdom
- Medical and Surgical Research Centre, IAHCP Education Academy, London, England, United Kingdom

Education:

Central London College, London, England, United Kingdom

- Chelmsford College of Further and Higher Education, Chelmsford, Essex, England, United Kingdom
- University of East London, Barking, Essex, England, United Kingdom
- Barts and The London School of Medicine and Dentistry, Queen Mary, University of London, England, United Kingdom

- Guys, Kings and St Thomas' Hospitals School of Medicine and Dentistry, Kings College, University of London, England, United Kingdom
- Faculty of Medicine and Dentistry, University of Dundee, Scotland, United Kingdom
- City University, London, England, United Kingdom
- University of East London, Barking, Essex, England, United Kingdom
- Higher Medial Institute, Ivan Petrovich Pavlov, Plovdiv, Bulgaria, Europe, currently Medical University, Plovdiv, Bulgaria, Europe
- Intitule of Medicine and Pharmacy, Carol Davila, Bucharest, Romania, currently Medical University – Carol Davila, Bucharest, Romania, Europe
- Other international Colleges, Universities and Institutions

Research and Professional Experience:

- Surgical Research - in all branches of surgery both for adult and paediatric populations.
- Medical Research - in all branches of medicine both for adult and paediatric populations.
- Epidemiology and Public Health Medicine
- General Practice, Family Medicine and Primary Care
- Medical and Healthcare Informatics
- Medical and Healthcare Education
- Hematology, Serology and Blood Transfusion
- General and Clinical Oncology Matters
- Global Health Issues
- Medical Innovations and application of new technology in health care
- Infectious diseases, parasitology and tropical diseases
- General Pathology, Clinical Pathology and Forensic Pathology

- Medical wiring, journalism, publications work and editing activities
- Evidence-based medicine and quality in healthcare
- Medical and Clinical Audit
- Research and developments in healthcare
- Dealing with Epidemics, pandemics and disasters
- Research methods in medicine and healthcare
- Research methods in Education and Medical Education
- Undergraduate medical education
- Postgraduate medical education
- Gastroenterology – both in adult and paediatric populations
- Histopathology and forensic medicine matters
- Obstetrics and Gynecology/Neonatology
- Comorbidity, Multi-morbidity, poly-morbidity ad poly-pharmacy issues
- Pediatrics and child health
- Coronavirus and COVID-19 issues
- Autoimmune diseases
- Chronic diseases
- Management of pain disorders and syndromes
- Diabetes and related issues
- Rheumatology and connective tissue diseases
- Dermatological diseases in adult and pediatric populations
- Rehabilitation in medicine and healthcare
- Neuroscience, Neurosurgery and Neurological issues
- Community Medicine
- Medical Prcatice in Developping Countries
- Surgical Methods of Human Diseases
- Diabetes and Endocrinolgy
- Nutition and effects of food on health
- Medical Emergencies and Disaster Medicine

Professional Appointments:

- Professor and Specialist in various and multiple medical, surgical and healthcare discipline (Professor of Medicine, Surgery, Epidemiology, Public Health, Global Health, Medical Education, Medical Informatics etc., at different institutions, academies and so on).
- Chief Medical Director
- Director of Surgical Services
- Director of Public Health
- Editor-in-Chief for various Scientific and Medical Journals, and Medical Publications Expert
- Chair of various Committees and Professional Groups at different institutions and organisations
- Expert and Consultant in various medical, surgical, healthcare specialties, and other originationsnal and management matters

Honors:

- Numerous awards, honor, scholarships and research grants from various institutions, agencies and organisations from 1981 to date
- Higher and honorary awards from different professional bodies from 1982 to date
- Life Membership and Fellowships of various organisations and Professional Bodies, from 1988 to date
- Royal College of General Practitioners, UK, International Travel Scholarship, 1994
- Many other honors and wards

More details of honors and awards of Professor Dr Daniella Kingsley-Godwin can be obtained by contacting daniellagodwin@ymail.com or dkingsley@iahcp.uk

Publications from the Last 3 Years:

2017:

1) Kingsley-Godwin. D., and Kingsley-Godwin. M. J. (2017). Diabetes Epidemics: A Challenge in the Changing World. *International Journal of Medicine.* 19 (1): 13-18.
2) Kingsley-Godwin D.E.C.C.O.H and Kingsley-Godwin. M. J. (2017). What is Minimally Invasive Surgery: Characteristics and Uses. *International Journal of Medicine.* 19(2):12-14.
3) Kingsley-Godwin D.E.C.C.O.H and Kingsley-Godwin. M. J. (2017). Minimally Invasive Surgery: Meeting the Challenges in Surgical Practice in the Changing World. *International Journal of Medicine.* 19 (3):21-27.
4) Kingsley-Godwin, Daniella. 2017. "Public Health Practice in the Past, Present and Future: The Dimensions of Health Policies from the European to National Perspectives – A Systematic Review." *Paper presented at the 1st International Conference on Public Health - "From European to National Health Policy,"* Faculty of Public Health, Sofia Medical University, Bulgaria, Europe, October 9 – 10.
5) Kingsley-Godwin D.E.C.C.O.H and Kingsley-Godwin. M. J. (2017). Clinical Benign Prostatic Hyperplasia: Evaluation of Epidemiological Issues, Diagnosis and Treatment Options. *The North and West London Journal of General Practice.* 9(2):20-28.
6) Kingsley-Godwin D.E.C.C.O.H and Kingsley-Godwin. M. J. (2017). Benign Prostatic Hyperplasia: A Common Problem in Society. *The North and West London Journal of General Practice.* 9(2):4-5.
7) Kingsley-Godwin D.E.C.C.O.H, Kingsley-Godwin. M. J. and Godwin. J (2017). Inflammation: Analysis of Characteristics. *The North and West London Journal of General Practice.* 9(2):6-7.

8) Kingsley-Godwin D.E.C.C.O.H and Kingsley-Godwin. M. J. (2017). From the Definition of Disease to the Explanation of the Disease Clinical Benign Prostatic Hyperplasia (BPH). *The North and West London Journal of General Practice.* 9(2):8-10.
9) Kingsley-Godwin D.E.C.C.O.H and Kingsley-Godwin. M. J. (2017). Benign Prostatic Hyperplasia: Management Matters in the Community. *The North and West London Journal of General Practice.* 9(2): 29-38.
10) Kingsley-Godwin. M. J., Kingsley-Godwin D.E.C.C.O.H, and Godwin. J. (2017). Understanding Disasters and Disaster Medicine: Exploring the Psychological and Ethical Issues. *The North and West London Journal of General Practice.* 9(1): 46-48.
11) Kingsley-Godwin D.E.C.C.O.H. (2017). Benign Prostatic Enlargement in General Practice: An Education Guide. *The North and West London Journal of General Practice.* 9(2): 11-16.

2018:

12) Kingsley-Godwin D.E.C.C.O.H. and Kingsley-Godwin M. J (2018). Understanding the Causes of Left Quadrant Abdominal Pain in Men and Women: Exploring Anatomy, Structure, Function, Pathophysiology, Diseases, Pains, Diagnosis, Treatments and Prevention – A Resource for General Practice and Primary Care. *The North and West London Journal of General Practice.* 10 (1):25-37.
13) Kingsley-Godwin D.E.C.C.O.H. and Kingsley-Godwin M. J (2018). Gastrointestinal Agents: Types, Drug Interactions and Side Effects, Including Liver-Tox Effect. *The North and West London Journal of General Practice*. 10 (1):20–24.
14) Kingsley-Godwin D.E.C.C.O.H. and Kingsley-Godwin M.J. (2018). Burkitt's Lymphoma: Examination of Aetiology, Pathophysiology, Histopathology, Treatment and Health Issues. *The North and West London Journal of General Practice.*10 (2) 2018:24-32.
15) Kingsley-Godwin D.E.C.C.O.H, Godwin. J, Kingsley-Godwin. M.J and Adams, S. (2018). Investigating Doxycline - Induced Oesphagitis:

A Clinical Study. *The North and West London Journal of General Practice*. 10(2):52-56.

16) Kingsley-Godwin D.E.C.C.O.H. and Kingsley-Godwin M. J, (2018). Foreign Bodies in the Ear, Nose and Throat in the Community: An Evaluation of Public Health and Epidemiological Issues – Towards the Production of Evidence-Based Guidelines for the Management of the Problem in the Community. *The North and West London Journal of General Practice* 10(1):59-60.
17) Kingsley-Godwin D.E.C.C.O.H. Godwin. J, Kingsley-Godwin M. J, and Adam. S, (2018). A Case of Tuberculous Lymphadenitis and Nodal Metastasis in Follicular Variant Papillary Carcinoma. *International Journal of Public Health Medicine.* 2(1):37-40.
18) Kingsley-Godwin D.E.C.C.O.H, Godwin. J, Kingsley-Godwin M. J, and Adam. S, (2018). A Case of Tuberculous Lymphadenitis and Nodal Metastasis in Follicular Variant Papillary Thyroid Carcinoma: A Confusing Encounter. *The North and West London Journal of General Practice* 10(2):39-42.
19) Kingsley-Godwin D.E.C.C.O.H. (2018). Effect of Autoimmunity on Society. *International Journal of Medicine*. 20(1):5-6.
20) Kingsley-Godwin D.E.C.C.O.H, Kingsley-Godwin M. J, and Godwin. J. (2018). Inflammation: Examination of Types, Processes and Management Issues in Health and Diseases. *International Journal of Medicine*. 20(1):33-52.
21) Kingsley-Godwin D.E.C.C.O.H. and Kingsley-Godwin M. J. (2018). Neurosarcoidosis: An Autoimmune Inflammatory Disease – Symptoms, Pathological Issues, Epidemiological Matters and Treatment. *International Journal of Medicine*. 20(1):57-62.
22) Kingsley-Godwin M. J, Kingsley-Godwin D.E.C.C.O.H and Godwin. J. (2018). Sarcoidosis: A Very Autoimmune Disease. *International Journal of Medicine*. 20(1):63-68.
23) Kingsley-Godwin D.E.C.C.O.H, Godwin. J. and Kingsley-Godwin M. J. (2018). Understanding the Impact of Sarcoidosis in the Community. *International Journal of Medicine*. 20(1):69-84.

24) Kingsley-Godwin D.E.C.C.O.H. and Kingsley-Godwin M. J. (2018). Rheumatoid Arthritis: A Serious Autoimmune Chronic Disease. *The North and West London Journal of General Practice.* 10(2):4-5.
25) Kingsley-Godwin D.E.C.C.O.H. (2018).Communication Skills: The Most Important Technique in Medicine. *Innovations in Health Professions Education.* 12(1):4-5.
26) Kingsley-Godwin D.E.C.C.O.H. (2018).Trends and Issues Affecting Education in Primary Care and Their Impact on General Practice Vocational Training: Systematic Review and Meta-Analysis. *Innovations in Health Professions Education.* 12(1):6-14.
27) Kingsley-Godwin D.E.C.C.O.H. and Godwin. J. (2018).Promoting Evidence-Based Practice in Healthcare: The Role of a New Distributed Health Information System. *Innovations in Health Professions Education.* 12(1):15-19.
28) Kingsley-Godwin. D. and Godwin. J. (2018). Multiprofessional Medical Emergency Teaching Using Telemedicine. *Innovations in Health Professions Education.* 12(1):40.
29) Godwin. J. and Kingsley-Godwin D.E.C.C.O.H. (2018).General Practitioners Knowledge of Legal Practicalities in Medicine: Evaluation of Disjunction, Errors, Uncertainties and Educational Needs. *Innovations in Health Professions Education.* 12(1):41.
30) Kingsley-Godwin D.E.C.C.O.H. and Kingsley-Godwin M. J. (2018). Lymphoma: History, Types, causes, Symptoms, Diagnosis, Treatment, Prognosis and Effects on Society. *The North and West London Journal of General Practice* 10(1):43-58.
31) Kingsley-Godwin D.E.C.C.O.H. and Kingsley-Godwin M. J. (2018). Lupus and Gastrointestinal Problems: The Role of Gastrointestinal Medications. *The North and West London Journal of General Practice* 10(1):4-5.

2019:

32) Kingsley-Godwin D.E.C.C.O.H and Kingsley-Godwin. M. J. (2019). Gastro-Oesophageal Reflux Disease in the Community. *The Primary Health Care Journal*. Volume 14(1):21-24.
33) Kingsley-Godwin D.E.C.C.O.H, Godwin. J. and Kingsley-Godwin. M. J. (2019). Analysis of Co-morbidity Issues, Public Health Matters and Educational Needs in Primary Care Mental Health. *International Journal of Primary Health Care*. 12 (1):16-23.
34) Kingsley-Godwin. D, Kingsley-Godwin. M. J. and Godwin. J. (2019). The Effect of Lyme Disease is Society. *International Journal of Medicine*. 21(1):4-5.
35) Kingsley-Godwin D.E.C.C.O.H, and Kingsley-Godwin. M. J. (2019). Systemic Lupus Erythematosus: A Serious Autoimmune Disease Pathological and Clinical Issues. *International Journal of Primary Health Care*. 12(2):20-34.
36) Kingsley-Godwin D.E.C.C.O.H and Kingsley-Godwin. M. J. (2019). Understanding Abdominal Wall Defects: Types and Characteristics. *Primary Health Care Journal*. 14(1): 29-35.
37) Kingsley-Godwin D.E.C.C.O.H and Kingsley-Godwin. M. J. (2019). Gastroschisis: A Rare and Important Paediatric Issue. *Primary Health Care Journal*. 14(1): 4-5.
38) Kingsley-Godwin D.E.C.C.O.H. (2019). Welcome to the North and West London Journal of General Practice (TNWLJGP). *The North and West London Journal of General Practice* 1(1):4.
39) Kingsley-Godwin D.E.C.C.O.H, and Godwin. J. (2019). Towards Efficient Global Health: Exploring the Health Threats in 2019. *International Journal of Primary Health Medicine.* 3(1): 9-12.
40) Kingsley-Godwin D.E.C.C.O.H, Godwin. J. and Kingsley-Godwin. M. J. (2019). Cardiac Surgery: Analysis of Ethical Dilemmas and Legal Issues. *Medical Law and Ethics Journal*. 13(1): 27-40.
41) Kingsley-Godwin D.E.C.C.O.H, Godwin. J. and Kingsley-Godwin. M. J. (2019). Robotic Surgery and Telesurgery Technology: Ethical

Dilemmas and Legal Practicalities. *Medical Law and Ethics Journal.* 13(1): 4-6.

42) Kingsley-Godwin D.E.C.C.O.H, Godwin. J. and Kingsley-Godwin. M. J. (2019). Principles of Disasters: Evaluation of Ethical Issues, Legal Practicalities and Complexity. *Medical Law and Ethics Journal.* 13(1):15-22.
43) Kingsley-Godwin D.E.C.C.O.H. and Kingsley-Godwin. M. J. (2019). Ethical Dilemma Examples – Analysing Moral Judgments. *Medical Law and Ethics Journal.* 13(1):23-26.
44) Kingsley-Godwin D.E.C.C.O.H, and Kingsley-Godwin. M. J. (2019). The Problem of Thalassaemia in the Community. *International Journal of Primary Health Care.* 12(1):4-6.
45) Kingsley-Godwin D.E.C.C.O.H, and Kingsley-Godwin. M. J. (2019). Haemoglobinopathies: Examination of Genetical and Diagnostic Issues. *International Journal of Primary Health Care.* 12(1):33-43.
46) Kingsley-Godwin D.E.C.C.O.H, and Kingsley-Godwin. M. J. (2019).Gastroschisis: A Rare and Important Paediatric Issue. *Primary Health Care Journal.* 14(1):4-5.
47) Kingsley-Godwin D.E.C.C.O.H. and Godwin. J. (2019). Towards Efficient Global Health: Exploring the Health Threats in 2019. *International Journal of Public health Medicine.* 3(1):9-12.
48) Kingsley-Godwin D.E.C.C.O.H, and Kingsley-Godwin. M. J. (2019). Systemic Lupus Erythematosus: A Serious Autoimmune Disease – Pathological and Clinical Issues. *International Journal of Primary Health Care.* 12(2):20-34.

2020:

49) Kingsley-Godwin. Daniella. 2020. "'Novel Coronavirus disease 2019': An emerging global pandemic." *Paper presented at the National scientific practical online conference with international participants – Nurses and midwives are the key resources in world health – Medical Faculty, Trakia University, Stara Zagora, Bulgaria, Europe*, October 29 – 30.

50) Kingsley-Godwin. Maria Jana, Kingsley-Godwin. Daniella, Godwin Joshua. 2020. "The Impact of Lime disease in the community." *Paper presented at the IAHCP Joint 39th International Online Medical Conference – Research and Innovations in Medical Practice and Education*, December 12 – 13.
51) Kingsley-Godwin. Daniella, Nencheva Elisaveta, Kingsley-Godwin. Maria Jana, Godwin Joshua, Georgieva Lidia, Georgiev Marin. 2020. "COVID-19: An emerging global pandemic of large magnitude." *Paper presented at the IAHCP Joint 39th International Online Medical Conference – Research and Innovations in Medical Practice and Education*, December 12 – 13.
52) Kingsley-Godwin. Daniella. 2020. "Examining Medical Innovations in the changing world: An interactive workshop." *Paper presented at the IAHCP Joint 39th International Online Medical Conference – Research and Innovations in Medical Practice and Education*, December 12–13.

For more information on the profile of Professor Dr Daniella E.C.C.O.H. Kingsley-Godwin, please click on the following link:

https://www.ijmjournal.org.uk/editorial-board-members/editorial-board-members-profiles/professor-dr-d-e-c-c-o-h-kingsley-godwin/

Maria Jana Kingsley-Godwin

Affiliation (s):

- London Medical Academy, London, England, United Kingdom
- Association of health Care Professionals and the International Association of Health Care Professionals (IAHCP) Society, London, England, United Kingdom
- Medical and Surgical Research Centre, IAHCP Education Academy

- Maria Jana (M.J.) Publications, London, England, United Kingdom

Education:

Stifford Clays Primary School, Grays, Essex, England, United Kingdom

- Park School for Girls, Ilford, Essex, England, United Kingdom
- Ilford Grammar School, Seven Kings, Ilford, Essex, England, United Kingdom
- St Annes College Grammar School, Lytham St Annes, Lancashire, England, United Kingdom
- IAHCP Education Academy, London, England, United Kingdom
- The Open University, Milton Keynes, England, United Kingdom
- Medical University – Plovdiv, Bulgaria, Europe

Research and Professional Experience:

- Surgical Research - in all branches of surgery both for adult and paediatric
- Medical Research - in all branches of medicine both for adult and paediatric
- Epidemiology and Public Health Medicine
- Medical and Healthcare Education
- Hematology, Serology and Blood Transfusion
- Clinical Oncology
- Global Health Issues
- Infectious diseases, parasitology and tropical diseases
- General Pathology Forensic pathology
- Medical wiring, journalism, publications work and editing activities

- Research and developments in healthcare
- Dealing with Epidemics, pandemics and disasters
- Research methods in medicine and healthcare
- Research methods in Education and Medical Education
- Gastroenterology – both in adult and paediatric populations
- Histopathology and forensic medicine matters
- Obstetrics and Gynecology/Neonatology
- Comorbidity, Multi-morbidity, poly-morbidity ad poly-pharmacy issues
- Pediatrics and child health
- Coronavirus and COVID-19 issues
- Autoimmune diseases
- Chronic diseases
- Management of pain disorders and syndromes
- Diabetes and related issues
- Rheumatology and connective tissue diseases
- Dermatological diseases
- Rehabilitation in medicine and healthcare
- Neurosurgery
- Neurology
- Neuroscience
- Human Anatomy
- Physiology and Pathophysiology
- Surgical Methods of Human Diseases

Professional Appointments:

- Medical Writer and Author
- Medical Healthcare Officer
- Medical and Healthcare Education Assessment Officer

Honors:

- Numerous awards, scholarships and research grants form various institutions, agencies and organisations from 2010 to date
- Membership of various organisations and professional bodies from 2016 to date

More details of honors and awards of Maria Jana Kingsley-Godwin can be obtained by contacting info@mariajana.co.uk or maria.jgodwin@gmail.com

Publications from the Last 3 Years:

2017:

1) Kingsley-Godwin. M. J. (2017). Echinococosis in the Community: Diagnosis and Management Issues. *The North and West London Journal of General Practice.* 9(1):19-22.
2) Kingsley-Godwin. D and Kingsley-Godwin. M. J. (2017). Diabetes Epidemics: A Challenge in the Changing World. *International Journal of Medicine.* 19(1):13-18.
3) Kingsley-Godwin. M. J. (2017). Lung Cancer: A Rising Problem in the Community – Clinical and Epidemiological Issues. *The North and West London Journal of General Practice.* 9(1):28-39.
4) Kingsley-Godwin. M. J. (2017). Food Insecurity and Chronic Diseases, and Severe Acute Malnutrition: Analysis of International Public Health Issues. *International Journal of Public Health Medicine.* 1:17-24.
5) Kingsley-Godwin. M. J. (2017).Video-Assisted Thoracoscopy (VATS): A Description of Characteristics. *International Journal of Medicine.* 19 (2):15-19.
6) Kingsley-Godwin. M. J. (2017). Laparoscopy: Analysis of Characteristics, Trends and Issues. *International Journal of Medicine.* 19(3):33-43.

7) Kingsley-Godwin D.E.C.C.O.H and Kingsley-Godwin. M.J. (2017).What is Minimally Invasive Surgery: Characteristics and Uses. *International Journal of Medicine*. 19(2):12-14.
8) Kingsley-Godwin D.E.C.C.O.H and Kingsley-Godwin. M.J. (2017). Minimally Invasive Surgery: Meeting the Challenges in Surgical Practice in the Changing World. *International Journal of Medicine*. 19(3):21-27.
9) Kingsley-Godwin. M. J. (2017). Examining the Epidemiological Issues of Eating Disorders in the Community. *International Journal of Public Health Medicine.* 19(1):5-7.
10) Kingsley-Godwin, Maria Jana. 2017. "Public Health issues in Chronic Diseases in the Community": A Resource for Health Policy Makers – Systematic Review. *Paper presented at the 1st International Conference on Public Health - "From European to National Health Policy," Faculty of Public Health, Sofia Medical University, Bulgaria, Europe*, October 9 – 10.
11) Kingsley-Godwin D.E.C.C.O.H and Kingsley-Godwin. M.J. (2017). Clinical Benign Prostatic Hyperplasia: Evaluation of Epidemiological Issues, Diagnosis and Treatment Options. *The North and West London Journal of General Practice.* 9(2):20-28.
12) Kingsley-Godwin D.E.C.C.O.H and Kingsley-Godwin. M.J. (2017). Benign Prostatic Hyperplasia: A Common Problem in Society. *The North and West London Journal of General Practice.* 9(2):4-5.
13) Kingsley-Godwin D.E.C.C.O.H, Kingsley-Godwin. M.J. and Godwin. J (2017). Inflammation: Analysis of Characteristics. *The North and West London Journal of General Practice.* 9(2):6-7.
14) Kingsley-Godwin D.E.C.C.O.H and Kingsley-Godwin. M. J. (2017). From the Definition of Disease to the Explanation of the Disease Clinical Benign Prostatic Hyperplasia (BPH). *The North and West London Journal of General Practice.* 9(2):8-10.
15) Kingsley-Godwin D.E.C.C.O.H and Kingsley-Godwin. M. J. (2017). Benign Prostatic Hyperplasia: Management Matters in the Community. *The North and West London Journal of General Practice.* 9(2): 29-38.

16) Kingsley-Godwin. M. J. (2017). Benign Prostatic Hyperplasia in the Community. *The North and West London Journal of General Practice.* 9(2): 50-51.
17) Kingsley-Godwin. M. J., Kingsley-Godwin D.E.C.C.O.H, and Godwin. J. (2017). Understanding Disasters and Disaster Medicine: Exploring the Psychological and Ethical Issues. *The North and West London Journal of General Practice.* 9(1): 46-48.
18) Kingsley-Godwin. M. J. (2017). Pneumonia: An Evaluation of Pathological, Clinical and Epidemiological Issues. *The North and West London Journal of General Practice*. 9(1):40-45.
19) Kingsley-Godwin. M. J. (2017). Neurosarcoidosis: Analysis of Features, Diagnosis and Treatment. *The North and West London Journal of General Practice*. 9(1):49-53.

2018:

20) Kingsley-Godwin M. J. (2018). Lupus and Gastrointestinal Problems: The Role of Gastrointestinal Medications. *The North and West London Journal of General Practice.* 10 (1):4-5.
21) Kingsley-Godwin D.E.C.C.O.H. and Kingsley-Godwin M. J. (2018). Understanding the Causes of Left Quadrant Abdominal Pain in Men and Women: Exploring Anatomy, Structure, Function, Pathophysiology, Diseases, Pains, Diagnosis, Treatments and Prevention – A Resource for General Practice and Primary Care. *The North and West London Journal of General Practice.* 10(1):25-37.
22) Kingsley-Godwin D.E.C.C.O.H. and Kingsley-Godwin M. J. (2018). Burkitt's Lymphoma: Examination of Aetiology, Pathophysiology, Histopathology, Treatment and Health Issues. *The North and West London Journal of General Practice*. 10(2):24 – 32.
23) Kingsley-Godwin D.E.C.C.O.H. and Kingsley-Godwin M. J (2018). Gastrointestinal Agents: Types, Drug Interactions and Side Effects, Including Liver-Tox Effect. *The North and West London Journal of General Practice*. 10(1):20 – 24.

24) Kingsley-Godwin D.E.C.C.O.H, Godwin. J, Kingsley-Godwin. M. J. and Adams, S. (2018). Investigating Doxycline - Induced Oesphagitis: A Clinical Study. *The North and West London Journal of General Practice.* 10(2):52-56.
25) Kingsley-Godwin. M. J. (2018). Using Robotic Surgical Technology in Improving Quality of Life and Saving the Lives of patients: Exploring the Expert Surgeons Opinions. *International Journal of Medicine.* 20(4):28-32.
26) Kingsley-Godwin D.E.C.C.O.H. and Kingsley-Godwin M. J. (2018). Foreign Bodies in the Ear, Nose and Throat in the Community: An Evaluation of Public Health and Epidemiological Issues – Towards the Production of Evidence-Based Guidelines for the Management of the Problem in the Community. *The North and West London Journal of General Practice.* 10(1):59-60.
27) Kingsley-Godwin. M. J. (2018). Robotic Surgery: Historical Perspectives and Characteristics. *International Journal of Medicine*. 20(4):25-27.
28) Kingsley-Godwin. M. J. (2018). Telesurgery: Analysis of Practicalities. *International Journal of Medicine.* 20(4):40-41.
29) Kingsley-Godwin. M. J. (2018). The Eye Lens: Anatomy, Diabetes and Complications. *The North and West London Journal of General Practice*. 10(1):38-42.
30) Kingsley-Godwin D.E.C.C.O.H, Godwin. J, Kingsley-Godwin M. J., and Adam. S, A. (2018). A Case of Tuberculous Lymphadenitis and Nodal Metastasis in Follicular Variant Papillary Carcinoma. *International Journal of Public Health Medicine.* 2(1):37-40.
31) Kingsley-Godwin M. J. (2018). Latent Tuberculosis Infection: An Evaluation of Eradication Initiatives. *International Journal of Public Health Medicine*. 2(2):30-35.
32) Kingsley-Godwin M. J. (2018). Chronic Diseases: Evaluation of Public Health Issues, Medical Matters and Surgical Perspectives. *International Journal of Public Health Medicine*. 2(2):36.

33) Kingsley-Godwin M. J. (2018). Autoimmune Diseases in the Changing World. *The North and West London Journal of General Practice*. 10(2):43-51.
34) Kingsley-Godwin M. J. (2018).Understanding Löfgren's Syndrome: An Autoimmune Phenomena. *The North and West London Journal of General Practice*. 10(2): 21-24.
35) Kingsley-Godwin D.E.C.C.O.H. Godwin. J., Kingsley-Godwin M. J., and Adam. S. (2018). A Case of Tuberculous Lymphadenitis and Nodal Metastasis in Follicular Variant Papillary Thyroid Carcinoma: A Confusing Encounter. *The North and West London Journal of General Practice* 10(2):39-42.
36) Kingsley-Godwin M. J. (2018). Evaluating the Impact of Autoimmunity in the Changing World. *International Journal of Medicine*. 20(1):13-22.
37) Kingsley-Godwin M. J. (2018). The Process of Autoimmunity: Exploring the Patters of Diseases, Diagnosis and Treatment. *International Journal of Medicine*. 20(1):23-32.
38) Kingsley-Godwin D.E.C.C.O.H, Kingsley-Godwin M. J., and Godwin. J. (2018). Inflammation: Examination of Types, Processes and Management Issues in Health and Diseases. *International Journal of Medicine*. 20(1):33-52.
39) Kingsley-Godwin D.E.C.C.O.H and Kingsley-Godwin M. J. (2018). Neurosarcoidosis: An Autoimmune Inflammatory Disease – Symptoms, Pathological Issues, Epidemiological Matters and Treatment. *International Journal of Medicine*. 20(1):57-62.
40) Kingsley-Godwin M. J, Kingsley-Godwin D.E.C.C.O.H and Godwin. J. (2018). Sarcoidosis: A Very Autoimmune Disease. *International Journal of Medicine*. 20(1):63-68.
41) Kingsley-Godwin D.E.C.C.O.H, Godwin. J. and Kingsley-Godwin M. J. (2018). Understanding the Impact of Sarcoidosis in the Community. *International Journal of Medicine*. 20(1):69-84.
42) Kingsley-Godwin D.E.C.C.O.H. and Kingsley-Godwin M. J. (2018).Rheumatoid Arthritis: A Serious Autoimmune Chronic Disease. *The North and West London Journal of General Practice* 10(2):4-5.

43) Kingsley-Godwin M. J. (2018). Glaucoma: A Serious Eye Disease in the Community. *The North and West London Journal of General Practice* 10(2):6-9.
44) Kingsley-Godwin M. J. (2018). Pulmonary Embolism: A Serious Health Issue – Time for More Effective Action in Patient Management. *The North and West London Journal of General Practice* 10(2):18-20.
45) Kingsley-Godwin. M. J. (2018). The Eye Lens: Anatomy, Structure, Functions and Clinical Significance. *The North and West London Journal of General Practice*. 10(2):33-38.
46) Kingsley-Godwin. M. J. (2018). The Eye Lens: Anatomy, Physiology, Diseases and Complications. *The North and West London Journal of General Practice*. 10(1):38-42.
47) Kingsley-Godwin D.E.C.C.O.H. and Kingsley-Godwin M. J. (2018). Lymphoma: History, Types, causes, Symptoms, Diagnosis, Treatment, Prognosis and Effects on Society. *The North and West London Journal of General Practice* 10(1):43-58.
48) Kingsley-Godwin D.E.C.C.O.H. and Kingsley-Godwin M. J. (2018). Lupus and Gastrointestinal Problems: The Role of Gastrointestinal Medications. *The North and West London Journal of General Practice* 10(1):4-5.

2019:

49) Kingsley-Godwin M. J. (2019). Anesthesiology: An Important Science and Medical Specialty. Guest Editorial. *The North and West London Journal of General Practice*. 11(1):4-5.
50) Kingsley-Godwin M. J. (2019). Dermatomyositis: Clinical Manifestations, Diagnosis, Pathological Issues, Treatment and Healthcare Matters. *The North and West London Journal of General Practice.* 11 (1):6-16.
51) Kingsley-Godwin M. J. (2019). Rehabilitation: Analysis of Characteristics, Types, Principles and Effects on Health and Wellbeing. *The North and West London Journal of General Practice*. 11(1):17-22.

52) Kingsley-Godwin M. J. (2019). Forensic Autopsy: An Evaluation of Principles and Practicalities. *The North and West London Journal of General Practice.* 11 (1):29-36.

53) Kingsley-Godwin M. J. (2019). Puerperium: Examination of the Physiological Principles, Management Matters, Postnatal Care and Health Issues, and Cultural Aspects of Postpartum. *The North and West London Journal of General Practice*. 11(2): 29-40.

54) Kingsley-Godwin D.E.C.C.O.H and Kingsley-Godwin. M. J. (2019). Gastro-Oesophageal Reflux Disease in the Community. *The Primary Health Care Journal*. 14(1):21-24.

55) Kingsley-Godwin D.E.C.C.O.H, Godwin. J. and Kingsley-Godwin. M. J. (2019). Analysis of Co-morbidity Issues, Public Health Matters and Educational Needs in Primary Care Mental Health. *International Journal of Primary Health Care*. 12 (1):16-23.

56) Kingsley-Godwin. M. J. (2019). Lyme Disease: An Emerging Infectious Disease in Temperate Regions of the World. *International Journal of Medicine*. 21(1):17-30.

57) Kingsley-Godwin. D, Kingsley-Godwin. M. J and Godwin. J. (2019).The Effect of Lyme Disease is Society. *International Journal of Medicine.* 21(1):4-5.

58) Kingsley-Godwin. M. J. (2019). Understanding Effects of Glaucoma in Society. *Primary Health Care Journal*. 14(2):6-18.

59) Kingsley-Godwin. M. J. (2019). Examination of Cranial Nerve Mononeuropathy: Anatomy, Functions, Disorder and Nerve Testing. *International Journal of Primary Health Care*.12 (2):41-50.

60) Kingsley-Godwin. M. J. (2019). Cranial Neuropathies: Anatomy, Types, Causes, Diagnosis, Treatment, Prevention and Health Issues. *International Journal of Primary Health Care*.12 (2):35-40.

61) Kingsley-Godwin. M. J. (2019). Cataracts: Analysis of Three Common Types – Their Causes, Symptoms, Prevention and Treatments. *International Journal of Primary Health Care.* 12 (2):6-8.

62) Kingsley-Godwin. M. J. (2019). Glaucoma: Symptoms, Treatment and Prevention in the Community. *International Journal of Primary Health Care*. 12(1):27-32.

63) Kingsley-Godwin D.E.C.C.O.H and Kingsley-Godwin. M. J. (2019). Understanding Abdominal Wall Defects: Types and Characteristics. *Primary Health Care Journal.* 14(1):29-35.
64) Kingsley-Godwin D.E.C.C.O.H and Kingsley-Godwin. M. J. (2019). Gastroschisis: A Rare and Important Paediatric Issue. *Primary Health Care Journal*. 14(1): 4-5.
65) Kingsley-Godwin D.E.C.C.O.H and Kingsley-Godwin. M. J. (2019). The Impacts of Cataract in the Community. *Primary Health Care Journal*. 14(1): 10-20.
66) Kingsley-Godwin. M. J. (2019). Tricyclic Antidepressant Overdose: Manifestations and Management Issues. *Primary Health Care Journal*. 14(2): 4-5.
67) Kingsley-Godwin. M. J. (2019). The Effects of Tricyclic Antidepressant in Society. *Primary Health Care Journal*. 14(2): 19-27.
68) Kingsley-Godwin. M. J. (2019). Tricyclic Antidepressant and Tricyclic Antidepressant: Analysis of Characteristics and Side Effects. *Primary Health Care Journal*. 14(2): 28-33.
69) Kingsley-Godwin. M. J. (2019). World Health Organisation New Release: Nine out of 10 People Worldwide Breathe Polluted Air, But More Countries are Taking Action. *International Journal of Public Health Medicine*. 3(1): 13-14.
70) Kingsley-Godwin D.E.C.C.O.H, Godwin. J. and Kingsley-Godwin. M. J. (2019). Cardiac Surgery: Analysis of Ethical Dilemmas and Legal Issues. *Medical Law and Ethics Journal*. 13(1): 27-40.
71) Kingsley-Godwin. M. J. (2019). Cardiopulmonary Bypass: Exploring Surgical Techniques and Practicalities. *International Journal of Primary Health Care*. 12(1): 47-56.
72) Kingsley-Godwin D.E.C.C.O.H, Godwin. J. and Kingsley-Godwin. M. J. (2019). Robotic Surgery and Telesurgery Technology: Ethical Dilemmas and Legal Practicalities. *Medical Law and Ethics Journal*. 13(1): 4-6.
73) Kingsley-Godwin D.E.C.C.O.H, Godwin. J. and Kingsley-Godwin. M. J. (2019). Principles of Disasters: Evaluation of Ethical Issues, Legal

Practicalities and Complexity. *Medical Law and Ethics Journal*. 13(1):15-22.

74) Kingsley-Godwin D.E.C.C.O.H. and Kingsley-Godwin. M. J. (2019). Ethical Dilemma Examples – Analysing Moral Judgments. *Medical Law and Ethics Journal*. 13(1):23-26.
75) Kingsley-Godwin D.E.C.C.O.H, and Kingsley-Godwin. M. J. (2019). The Problem of Thalassaemia in the Community. *International Journal of Primary Health Care*. 12(1):4-6.
76) Kingsley-Godwin D.E.C.C.O.H, and Kingsley-Godwin. M. J. (2019). Haemoglobinopathies: Examination of Genetical and Diagnostic Issues. *International Journal of Primary Health Care*. 12(1):33-43.
77) Kingsley-Godwin. M. J. (2019). Hospital in the Home: An Australian State Perspective. *International Journal of Primary Health Care*. 12(1):44-46.
78) Kingsley-Godwin D.E.C.C.O.H, and Kingsley-Godwin. M. J. (2019).Gastroschisis: A Rare and Important Paediatric Issue. *Primary Health Care Journal*. 14(1):4-5.
79) Kingsley-Godwin D.E.C.C.O.H, and Kingsley-Godwin. M. J. (2019). Systemic Lupus Erythematosus: A Serious Autoimmune Disease – Pathological and Clinical Issues. *International Journal of Primary Health Care*. 12(2):20-34.

2020:

80) Kingsley-Godwin. Maria Jana. 2020. "'Issues in Scoliosis': Chronic Orthopaedic Manifestations in the Community." *Paper presented at the National scientific practical online conference with international participants – Nurses and midwives are the key resources in world health – Medical Faculty*, Trakia University, Stara Zagora, Bulgaria, Europe, October 29–30.
81) Kingsley-Godwin. Maria Jana, Kingsley-Godwin. Daniella, Godwin Joshua. 2020. "The Impact of Lime disease in the community." *Paper presented at the IAHCP Joint 39th International Online Medical*

Conference – Research and Innovations in Medical Practice and Education, December 12–13.

82) Kingsley-Godwin. Daniella, Nencheva Elisaveta, Kingsley-Godwin. Maria Jana, Godwin Joshua, Georgieva Lidia, Georgiev Marin. 2020. "COVID-19: An emerging global pandemic of large magnitude." *Paper presented at the IAHCP Joint 39th International Online Medical Conference – Research and Innovations in Medical Practice and Education*, December 12 – 13.

For more information on the profile of Maria Jana Kingsley-Godwin, please visit her website at:
www.mariajana.co.uk

Joshua Kingsley-Godwin

Affiliation (s):

- London Medical Academy, London, England, United Kingdom
- Association of health Care Professionals and the International Association of Health Care Professionals (IAHCP) Society, London, England, United Kingdom
- Medical and Surgical Research Centre, IAHCP Education Academy, London, England, United Kingdom
- Santa Maria College of the Association of Health Care Professionals, London, England, United Kingdom

Education:

- Chelmsford College of Further and Higher Education, Chelmsford, Essex, England, United Kingdom
- University of East London, Barking, Essex, England, United Kingdom

- Guys, Kings and St Thomas' Hospitals School of Medicine and Dentistry, Kings College, University of London, England, United Kingdom

Research and Professional Experience:

- Surgical Research - in all branches of surgery both for adult and paediatric
- Medical Research - in all branches of medicine both for adult and paediatric
- Epidemiology and Public Health Medicine
- General Practice, Family Medicine and Primary Care
- Medical and Healthcare Informatics
- Medical and Healthcare Education
- Global Health Issues
- Medical Law
- Medical Ethics
- Medical wiring, journalism, publications work and editing activities
- Evidence-based medicine and quality in healthcare
- Research and developments in healthcare
- Dealing with Epidemics, pandemics and disasters
- Research Methods in medicine and healthcare
- Research Methods in Education and Medical Education
- Undergraduate medical education
- Postgraduate medical education
- Comorbidity, Multi-morbidity, poly-morbidity ad poly-pharmacy issues
- Coronavirus and COVID-19 issues
- Diabetes and related issues
- Rehabilitation in medicine and healthcare

Professional Appointments:

- Professor of Medical Law and Ethics
- Director of Public Health
- Editor-in-Chief for Medical Law and Ethics Journal

Honors:

- Numerous awards, scholarships and research grants form various institutions, agencies and organisations from 1990 to date
- Higher and honorary awards from different professional bodies from 1992 to date
- Fellowships of various organisations and professional bodies, from 1988 to date

Publications from the Last 3 Years:

2017:

1) Godwin, Joshua. 2017. "'Understanding Manmade Diseases in the Changing World': Towards the Development of an Efficient Knowledge-based Media for Effective Management of Diseases." *Paper presented at the 1st International Conference on Public Health - "From European to National Health Policy," Faculty of Public Health, Sofia Medical University, Bulgaria, Europe*, October 9 – 10.
2) Kingsley-Godwin D.E.C.C.O.H, Kingsley-Godwin. M.J. and Godwin. J (2017). Inflammation: Analysis of Characteristics. *The North and West London Journal of General Practice.* 9(2):6-7.
3) Kingsley-Godwin. M. J., Kingsley-Godwin D.E.C.C.O.H, and Godwin. J. (2017). Understanding Disasters and Disaster Medicine: Exploring the Psychological and Ethical Issues. *The North and West London Journal of General Practice.* 9(1): 46-48.

2018:

4) Kingsley-Godwin D.E.C.C.O.H, Godwin. J, Kingsley-Godwin. M. J, and Adams, S. (2018). Investigating Doxycline - Induced Oesphagitis: A Clinical Study. *The North and West London Journal of General Practice.* 10(2):52-56.
5) Kingsley-Godwin D.E.C.C.O.H. Godwin. J, Kingsley-Godwin M. J, and Adam. S, A. (2018). A Case of Tuberculous Lymphadenitis and Nodal Metastasis in Follicular Variant Papillary Carcinoma. *International Journal of Primary Health Medicine.* 2(1):37-40.
6) Kingsley-Godwin D.E.C.C.O.H, Godwin. J, Kingsley-Godwin M. J, and Adam. S, (2018). A Case of Tuberculous Lymphadenitis and Nodal Metastasis in Follicular Variant Papillary Thyroid Carcinoma: A Confusing Encounter. *The North and West London Journal of General Practice* 10(2):39-42.
7) Kingsley-Godwin D.E.C.C.O.H, Kingsley-Godwin M. J, and Godwin. J. (2018). Inflammation: Examination of Types, Processes and Management Issues in Health and Diseases. *International Journal of Medicine*. 20(1):33-52.
8) Kingsley-Godwin M. J, Kingsley-Godwin D.E.C.C.O.H, and Godwin. J. (2018). Sarcoidosis: A Very Autoimmune Disease. *International Journal of Medicine*. 20(1):63-68.
9) Kingsley-Godwin D.E.C.C.O.H, Godwin. J. and Kingsley-Godwin M. J. (2018). Understanding the Impact of Sarcoidosis in the Community. *International Journal of Medicine*. 20(1):69-84.
10) Kingsley-Godwin D.E.C.C.O.H. and Godwin. J. (2018).Promoting Evidence-Based Practice in Healthcare: The Role of a New Distributed Health Information System. *Innovations in Health Professions Education.* 12(1):15-19.
11) Kingsley-Godwin. D. and Godwin. J. (2018). Multiprofessional Medical Emergency Teaching Using Telemedicine. *Innovations in Health Professions Education.* 12(1):40.

12) Godwin. J. and Kingsley-Godwin D.E.C.C.O.H. (2018).General Practitioners Knowledge of Legal Practicalities in Medicine: Evaluation of Disjunction, Errors, Uncertainties and Educational Needs. *Innovations in Health Professions Education.* 12(1):41.

2019:

13) Godwin. J. (2019). The Royal of Rehabilitation Nurses in the Management of Patients' Illnesses in the Community. *The North and West London Journal of General Practice*. 11(1):23-28.
14) Kingsley-Godwin D.E.C.C.O.H, Godwin. J. and Kingsley-Godwin. M. J. (2019). Analysis of Co-morbidity Issues, Public Health Matters and Educational Needs in Primary Care Mental Health. *International Journal of Primary Health Care*. 12(1):16-23.
15) Kingsley-Godwin. D, Kingsley-Godwin. M. J and Godwin. J. (2019). The Effect of Lyme Disease is Society. *International Journal of Medicine*. 21(1):4-5.
16) Godwin. J. (2019). Disaster and Emergency Medicine- A Conceptual Introduction. *International Journal of Public Health Medicine*. 3(1): 4-6.
17) Kingsley-Godwin D.E.C.C.O.H, and Godwin. J. (2019). Towards Efficient Global Health: Exploring the Health Threats in 2019. *International Journal of Public Health Medicine*. 3(1): 9-12.
18) Kingsley-Godwin D.E.C.C.O.H, Godwin. J. and Kingsley-Godwin. M. J. (2019). Cardiac Surgery: Analysis of Ethical Dilemmas and Legal Issues. *Medical Law and Ethics Journal*. 13(1): 27-40.
19) Godwin. J (2019). Improving Public Health Outcomes with Electronic Health Records. *Medical Law and Ethics Journal*. 13(1): 7.
20) Kingsley-Godwin D.E.C.C.O.H, Godwin. J. and Kingsley-Godwin. M. J. (2019). Principles of Disasters: Evaluation of Ethical Issues, Legal Practicalities and Complexity. *Medical Law and Ethics Journal*. 13(1):15-22.

21) Godwin. J. (2019). Living with Manmade Disease: Evaluating Good Health. *International Journal of Public Health Care*. 12(2):4-5.
22) Godwin. J. (2019). Is Manmade Disease a Product of Direct or Deliberate Intervention by an Individual Lifestyle or Governments' Action? *The North and West London Journal of General Practice*. 9(1):4.
23) Godwin. J. (2019). Disaster and Emergency Medicine- A Conceptual Introduction. *International Journal of Public Health Medicine*. 3(1):4-5.
24) Kingsley-Godwin D.E.C.C.O.H. and Godwin. J. (2019). Towards Efficient Global Health: Exploring the Health Threats in 2019. *International Journal of Public Health Medicine*. 3(1):9-12.
25) Kingsley-Godwin D.E.C.C.O.H, Godwin. J. and Kingsley-Godwin. M. J. (2019). Robotic Surgery and Telesurgery Technology: Ethical Dilemmas and Legal Practicalities. *Medical Law and Ethics Journal*. 13(1): 4-6.

2020:

26) Godwin Joshua. 2020. "The role of rehabilitation nurses in the management of patients in the community." *Paper presented at the National scientific practical online conference with international participants – Nurses and midwives are the key resources in world health – Medical Faculty, Trakia University, Stara Zagora, Bulgaria, Europe*, October 29–30.
27) Godwin Joshua. 2020. "Rehabilitation following the impact of COVID-19." *Paper presented at the IAHCP Joint 39th International Online Medical Conference – Research and Innovations in Medical Practice and Education*, December 12–13.

28) Kingsley-Godwin. Maria Jana, Kingsley-Godwin. Daniella, Godwin Joshua. 2020. "The Impact of Lime disease in the community." *Paper presented at the IAHCP Joint 39th International Online Medical Conference – Research and Innovations in Medical Practice and Education*, December 12–13.

29) Kingsley-Godwin. Daniella, Nencheva Elisaveta, Kingsley-Godwin. Maria Jana, Godwin Joshua, Georgieva Lidia, Georgiev Marin. 2020. "COVID-19: An emerging global pandemic of large magnitude." *Paper presented at the IAHCP Joint 39th International Online Medical Conference – Research and Innovations in Medical Practice and Education*, December 12–13.

In: Burkitt Lymphoma
Editor: Douglas V. Berthelot
ISBN: 978-1-68507-071-7

Chapter 2

BURKITT LYMPHOMA IN PATIENTS WITH PRIMARY IMMUNODEFICIENCY DISORDERS

***Zeinab Afify*[1,*] *and Oussama Abla*[2]**
[1]Division of Hematology/Oncology, Department of Pediatrics, University of Utah, Salt Lake City, Utah, US
[2]Division of Hematology/Oncology, Department of Pediatrics, Hospital for Sick Children, Toronto, Ontario, Canada

ABSTRACT

Mature B cell Non-Hodgkin lymphoma (B-NHL) including Burkitt lymphoma (BL) and diffuse large B cell lymphoma (DLBCL) are among the most common malignancies associated with primary immune deficiency disorders (PIDs). Unlike sporadic BL, PIDs associated B-NHL are commonly Epstein Barr virus (EBV) driven.

There is a wide spectrum of PIDs associated with BL resulting in unique features with each association. For example, patients with X-linked lymphoproliferative disease type 1 (XLP1) are at particularly high risk of developing multiple lymphomas. Other PIDs are also chromosome instability syndromes, such as ataxia telangiectasia (AT) and Bloom

* Corresponding Author's E-mail: zeinab.afify@imail.org.

Syndrome (BS). In these syndromes, chemotherapy, if not modified, confers a high risk of severe morbidity and mortality.

Patients with PIDs are routinely excluded from clinical trials of B-NHL, therefore, limited data are available regarding potential differences in lymphoma biology, risk factors, optimal treatment strategies, and outcome. The prognosis of these patients is overall poor due to increased treatment-related toxicities and/or treatment refractoriness. These patients require modifications of certain components of intensive therapy with careful attention to supportive care, but there is no consensus with regard to the optimal treatment strategies.

Historically, many patients with PIDs associated lymphomas were treated with minimal or modified reduced-intensity therapy. The incorporation of novel targeted agents like monoclonal antibodies into less intensive standard chemotherapy regimens may help address the challenges of treatment-associated toxicities and refractory disease. Immunotherapies, however, bring uncertainties of the quality and duration of subsequent immune reconstitution.

Despite the rarity of these cases, every pediatric and lymphoma oncologist will face these challenges in their career. After 3 real world case presentations, this chapter will review the spectrum, unique characteristics and special management considerations when BL develops in specific subgroups of patients with PIDs.

Keywords: Burkitt lymphoma, primary immune deficiency disorders, chromosome instability syndromes, ataxia telangiectasia, Bloom syndrome, Wiscott Aldrich syndrome

1. INTRODUCTION

Cancer occurs with a higher incidence rate and manifests earlier in life in patients with primary immunodeficiency disorders (PIDs) than in the general population [1]. It is the second-leading cause of death after infection in both children and adults with PIDs [2-4]. Increased awareness of clinicians, coupled with advances in genetics, has led to a surge in the diagnosis of malignancies associated with PIDs [4].

Furthermore, the impact of PIDs-associated malignancies has recently increased in parallel with improved survival and longevity of patients with PIDs [5]. Despite this, immunodeficient patients who develop malignancy including lymphoma, have a worse prognosis compared to immunocompetent individuals with histologically similar malignancies [6, 7].

The high incidence and the pattern of malignancies in patients with PID is not explained by an increased tumor immune escape alone. Based on recent studies of malignancies in large PIDs cohorts, a large part of tumor predisposition in patients with PIDs is derived from the same molecular defect as the immunodeficiency itself. Lymphomas in particular are mostly restricted to tissue types bearing the same molecular defect that underlies the PIDs, such as syndromes of DNA repair defects, or immune cell–specific maturation or functional defects, thus suggesting a cell-intrinsic oncogenic basis [1].

Non-Hodgkin lymphoma (NHL) is the most common malignancy in patients with PIDs, with B-NHL as the leading subtype. Unlike B-NHL in immunocompetent (IC) patients, Burkitt lymphoma (BL) is less common than diffuse large B cell lymphoma (DLBCL) in patients with PIDs [5, 8]. In children, these 2 NHL subtypes are equally aggressive, treated with identical chemotherapy or chemoimmunotherapy regimens, and have the same favorable outcome [9-14]. Most reports of B-NHL in patients with PIDs combine the 2 subtypes. Therefore, in this chapter we will review the reported treatments administered and outcomes of a combination of BL and DLBCL, often without providing BL specific data. We will focus on special characteristics and mechanisms of lymphomagenesis in the most common types of PIDs associated with BL (PID-BL). Clinical cases will be presented to illustrate some of the challenges posed by the increased risk of treatment-related morbidity and mortality, risk of second lymphomas and other unique long-term complications of therapy.

2. Clinical Cases

2.1. Case-1 [15]

A seven-year-old male refugee from sub-Saharan Africa presented with a croupy cough and a mediastinal mass and was diagnosed with Epstein Barr Virus (EBV) positive BL, stage III, risk group B according to FAB-LMB clinical risk group stratification. He received full dose chemotherapy per standard FAB/LMB Children's Cancer Group protocol CCG 5961, without rituximab. After receiving the first intensive chemotherapy cycle consisting of cyclophosphamide, doxorubicin, high dose methotrexate, vincristine, prednisone, and intrathecal chemotherapy, he suffered from grade 4 myelosuppression and mucositis, both were unusually prolonged and resulted in delay in future cycles. He developed impaired cardiac function that required inotropic medications. Signs and symptoms of chronic lung disease developed after end of therapy and he was found to have ataxia telangiectasia (AT). The patient continued to be in complete remission (CR), but died of complications of chronic lung disease 18 months after end of therapy. In retrospect, one of his brothers had ataxia and was subsequently also diagnosed with AT.

2.2. Case 2 [16]

A 4-year-old male was diagnosed with appendicular BL, stage II, clinical risk group B. He was successfully treated with chemotherapy CCG 5961 protocol without dose reduction or treatment modifications. At age 8 years he developed ileocecal DLBCL. The 2 lymphomas were EBV negative and were clonally distinct. Genetic predisposition was suspected. Further genetic testing of the patient was positive for SH2D1A gene mutation which was also positive in several male relatives. He was successfully treated with the same regimen and underwent matched unrelated allogeneic hematopoietic stem cell transplantation (allo-HSCT). He remains in remission for 2 years and 2 months after allo-HSCT.

3. Epidemiology

Primary immunodeficiency disorders are associated with a markedly increased risk of cancer, particularly NHL. This association has been noted for many years [17-25], has been confirmed by single-center studies, and from data collected in established registries [26-35]. Overall 4–25% of patients with PIDs develop cancer. This is much higher in certain subtypes of PIDs such as chromosome instability disorders [2, 5, 27]. The increasing life expectancy in patients with PIDs, is likely to result in increased incidence of malignancies as these patients get older [4, 5]. Table 1 shows the incidence of PIDs in the general population and the overall risk of patients with PIDs to develop malignancy.

3.1. Data from Large PIDs Registries

Over the last decade, data from large PIDs registries provided current cancer incidence data in PIDs [32, 35]. Further establishing the association recognized already in the early 1970's [23]. An excess of lymphoma in specific PIDs populations principally drove this increased incidence, with no increased risk of the most common solid tumors [35]. Data from international registries of PIDs show that lymphoma is the most frequent cancer with NHL taking the lead [32, 35]. Taken as a whole, most large registries show 8-11-fold increased risk of lymphoma in patients with all PIDs combined [26, 32, 35]. Non-Hodgkin lymphoma is the predominant malignancy in a number of PIDs, including common variable immunodeficiency (CVID), ataxia telangiectasia (AT), Wiskott Aldrich syndrome (WAS), among others [4, 26, 35], with B-NHL as the predominant NHL subtype [8, 27].

Table 1. Classification of PIDs commonly associated with NHL [4, 5, 8, 23, 24, 33, 35, 54, 64, 70, 73]

Category of PID	PID	Genetic defect	Inheritance	Incidence of PID	Risk X fold (or prevalence)			% cancer*
					Cancer	Lymphoma	NHL	
All PIDs				1:4000	1.4 - 2.3	8-11	NR	4-25%
Chromosome instability syndromes	AT	ATM	AR	1:100,000	100	252-750	NR	10-33%
	NBS	NBS1	AR	1:1,000,000	61	252	200-700	42%
	BS	BLM	AR	1:100,000-250,000	50	NR	250	50%
Immunodeficiency with congenital thrombocytopenia	WAS	WAS	XL	1;100,000 – 1:1,000,000	100	(4.1%)	NR	13–23%
Predominantly antibody deficiencies	CVID	Unknown	Variable	1:25,000 – 1: 50,000	5–12	15	NR	13.1%
Disorders of immune dysregulation	ALPS	TNFRSF6	AD or AR	Unknown Several hundred cases reported	100	NR	12	NR
	XLP1	SH2D1A	XL	1:3,000,000 males	2.3	(14.3-33%)	51 (53% of B-NHL are BL)	14.3-33% develop lymphoma

*Percent of individuals who develop cancer.

PIDs: Primary immunodeficiency disorders; NHL: Non-Hodgkin lymphoma; AT: ataxia telangiectasia; NBS: Nijmegen breakage syndrome; BS: Bloom syndrome; WAS: Wiskott Aldrich syndrome; CVID: common variable immunodeficiency; ALPS: autoimmune lymphoproliferative syndrome; XLP1: X-linked lymphoproliferative disorder; AR: autosomal recessive; AD: autosomal dominant; XL: X- linked; NR: not reported.

3.2. Age and Gender Distribution

Gender distribution in patients with PIDs who develop cancer is almost equal in several studies, with a slight increase in males in some [27, 32, 33, 35]. Overall, males with PIDs have a higher increased risk of lymphoma (10 fold in males and 8-fold in females). This can partly be explained by X- linked PIDs [35]. However, this gender distribution is variable among studies, and the type of lymphoma. Two recent studies found a more striking male predominance in patients with PIDs-associated NHL. The first, a study of 690 patients with PIDs from a large pediatric center in Italy found a male predominance among patients with PIDs and NHL (22 males and 16 females) [27]. The second study by Attarbaschi et al., found a male predominance (65%) in children and adolescents with NHL who have predisposing conditions including PIDs [8].

There are no available age-specific data for B-NHL and BL in patients with PIDs. The age at developing lymphoma varies depending on the underlying PID. In a study by Maffeis et al., of 690 patients with PIDs, the mean age at cancer diagnosis was 32.75 years in patients with CVID, an immunodeficiency that usually manifests itself in adulthood. This is in contrast to patients with combined immunodeficiencies (CID) where the mean age at cancer diagnosis was 9 years [27].

3.3. Burkitt Lymphoma in Patients with PIDs

Despite data from large registries, there is scarce systematic data on the spectrum of NHL subtypes associated with PIDs, their clinical characteristics and outcome [8]. The most detailed recent data were provided by two studies in patients with PIDs associated NHL [8, 27].

A multinational study of 213 pediatric patients with predisposing conditions including PIDs, was conducted by 2 childhood NHL consortia, the European Intergroup for Childhood NHL (EICNHL) and the international Berlin-Frankfurt-Münster (i-BFM) Study Group (SG).

There were 103 patients with PIDs who developed NHL. The most frequent were PIDs associated with chromosome instability; AT and Nijmegen breakage syndrome (NBS) followed by Wiscott Aldrich syndrome (WAS), X-linked lymphoproliferative disorder (XLP1), and CVID. Fourteen of the 55 (25%) patients with B-NHL in this study had BL [8].

In the study by Maffies et al., NHL was the most frequent tumor (16 of 33 of the hematologic malignancies: ten had B-NHL (8 had DLBCL, and two had BL). Of the two patients with Burkitt lymphoma one had CVID and the other had AT [27]. Table-2 summarizes cases of PID-BL reported in large studies and in individual case reports.

In immunocompetent (IC) children, DLBCL and BL subtypes are equally aggressive, treated on identical chemotherapy or chemoimmunotherapy regimens and have similar favorable outcomes with optimal supportive care measures [9-14]. Interestingly in IC children, BL is more common than DLBCL [37, 38], and the reason for the much smaller number of BL compared to DLBCL in patients with PIDs is unclear. However, their outcome could be similar, but this remains uncertain due to the very small number of reported PID-BL cases and the scarcity of published data about treatment and outcome in these subgroups [8, 27, 36, 39-41]. On the other hand, BL in IC adults is rare and more aggressive than most DLBCL [42, 43]. It is unclear from the published literature how many adults with PIDs develop BL, since most registries and reports combined children and adults [26, 32, 35]. The male gender predominance in IC-BL patients, may be present in BL associated with PIDs, but this is also uncertain due to the limited BL specific data available from PIDs registries, cooperative groups, large institution studies and individual case reports.

Table 2. Burkitt lymphomas reported in patients with PIDs over last 20 years

Ref./Year	PID	Number B-NHL	Number BL		Gender/ Age in years	Location	Treatment of BL	Outcome in years*
Registries, cooperative groups and large institution studies								
[73] 2001	ALPS	6	ALPS	2	M/ 50 F / 17	Omental mass Abdomen	Chemotherapy, NR COP	CR 4 CR 1
[80] 2009	NBS	8	NBS	2	M/ 9.1 F / 5.8	NR	LMB-89, 50–85% dose LMB-89, 80–100%	CR 5.4 CR 6.2
[36] 2011	AT NBS	20	AT NBS	2 2	M/ 16.3 M/ 7.7 M/ 5.9 M/ 4.9	NR	NHL-BFM 04 NHL-BFM 04 NHL-BFM 95 NHL-BFM 90	Died, lung disease CR 2.7 CR 6.5 CR 6.5
[39] 2014	AT	5	AT	1	M/ 11	BM, CNS	LMB-89	DOD
[105] 2015	All	8	WAS XLP1	1 1	M/ 6.3 M/ 6	Abdomen, bowel Abdomen, bowel	NHL-BFM NHL-BFM95	Died of 2nd BL CR 5.7
[29] 2015	All	28	AT	2	M/ 11 M/ 8	Pharynx, cervical LN Pharynx	AIEOP LNH-97, 20% reduction alkylating agents AIEOP LNH-97, 50% reduction MTX	CR 1.2 CR 2
[8] 2016	All	55	AT NBS XLP1 WAS	6 2 5 1	NR	NR	Multiple international cooperative groups regimens	NR
[27] 2019	All	10	CVID AT	1 1	NR	NR	NR	NR

Table 2. (Continued)

Ref./Year	PID	Number B-NHL	Number BL		Gender/ Age in years	Location	Treatment of BL	Outcome in years*
Case reports								
[41] 2006	WAS	1	WAS	1	M/ 12	Ileocecal	NR	NR
[104] 2013	AT	1	AT	1	F/ 11	Ovary	rituximab, FAB/LMB	NR
[40] 2016	BS	1	BS	1	M/ 5	Abdomen, liver	LMB	DOD 1.1
[69] 2016	XLP1	1	XLP1	1	M/ 6	Abdomen	FAB/LMB	CR 7, DOC of 2nd BL
[103] 2016	CVID	1	CVID	1	F/ 11	Inguinal LN	CHOP	CR 5, 2nd lymphoma
[79] 2017	BS	1	BS	1	M/11	Larynx, Mediastinum	LMB, vincristine, prednisone, rituximab	CR 4
[16] 2021	XLP1	1	XLP1	1	M/3.9	Ileocecal	FAB/LMB	CR 4, 2nd BL: CR 2

*Number of years in remission; NR: not reported; CR: complete remission, DOD: died of disease; DOC: died of complications; LN: lymph nodes; PID: Primary immunodeficiency; NHL: Non-Hodgkin lymphoma; BL: Burkitt lymphoma; AT: ataxia telangiectasia; NBS: Nijmegen breakage syndrome; BS: Bloom syndrome; WAS: Wiskott Aldrich syndrome; CVID: common variable immunodeficiency; ALPS: autoimmune lymphoproliferative syndrome; XLP1: X-linked lymphoproliferative disorder; COP: cyclophosphamide, vincristine, prednisolone; R-CHOP: rituximab, cyclophosphamide, doxorubicin, vincristine, prednisolone.

4. LYMPHOMAGENESIS IN IMMUNE DEFICIENCY DISORDERS

4.1. Cancer Immune Surveillance in Immune Deficiency Disorders

Defective immune surveillance is considered a major factor in the complex relationship between underlying immune deficiency, viral infections and the development of cancer in people with PIDs [3-5, 44]. The most common cancer subtype in immunodeficient patients is lymphoma, an immune system-related malignancy [3, 5]. However, not all these lymphomas are associated with infectious agents such as EBV. Therefore, a defect in immune surveillance may be in the identification and or elimination of cells with abnormalities of proliferation, function and/or apoptosis and more than just the inability to properly control infections [1, 7, 45].

4.2. EBV and PIDs-Associated Lymphoma

Infection with oncogenic viruses, results in the transduction of copies of the viral genome into cellular genes that can activate proto-oncogenes, inactivate tumor suppressor cells or stimulate growth factors. Epstein Barr virus infection causes polyclonal activation and proliferation of B-cells. Immunity against this virus is primarily carried out by $CD8^+$ cytotoxic T-cells and to a lesser degree by other immune mechanisms such as humoral responses or natural killer cell activity [30]. It is well known that patients with congenital and acquired immunodeficiency are more prone to develop lymphoproliferative disease associated with EBV, or less frequently with other viral infections [4, 30, 45]. Epstein Barr virus in particular appears to be an important co-factor for the development of PIDs-associated lymphomas and is found in 30–60% of cases [27]. Primary immune deficiency disorders with T-cell dysfunction are expected to be particularly susceptible to EBV-related lymphomas, due to reduction of EBV-specific CD8 T cells [27, 30].

4.3. Mechanisms of Lymphomagenesis in PIDs

Despite strong support for the physiologic role of tumor immune surveillance, the incidence and pattern of malignancies in patients with PIDs do not reflect an increased tumor immune escape alone as a causative mechanism. There is growing evidence that the predilection for developing cancer in immunodeficient hosts may not be a specific immune defect in the recognition of viral specific antigens, but a defect in immune surveillance necessary for elimination of cells with abnormalities in proliferation, function and/or apoptosis [1, 45]. Lymphoma, the major malignancy associated with PIDs, commonly occurs in association with PIDs characterized by immune cell–specific maturation or functional defects, thus suggesting a cell-intrinsic oncogenic basis. Most PIDs associated lymphomas appear to be restricted to tissue types bearing the same molecular defect that underlies the PIDs, as in lymphomas associated with syndromes of DNA repair defects [1].

Several mechanisms can explain the association between PIDs and malignancies. These mechanisms have been broadly categorized into intrinsic and extrinsic to the defective immune cells. Intrinsic factors include impaired cell development, intra-cellular signaling, chromosome instability, and impaired immune surveillance, while extrinsic factors consist of chronic infection and tissue inflammation. Therefore, non-immune mechanisms exist to prevent neoplastic transformation and include DNA repair, epigenetic mechanisms, intracellular and intercellular surveillance. The complexity of the origin of lymphomatous transformation in PIDs is partly related to the heterogeneity of the underlying conditions [1]. Table-3 outlines mechanisms of lymphomagenesis in most common PIDs associated with lymphoma.

5. Primary Immune Deficiency Disorders Commonly Associated with Lymphoma

Table-1 outlines the most common PIDs associated with lymphoma and their incidence.

5.1. Chromosome Instability Syndromes

5.1.1. Ataxia Telangiectasia (AT)

Patients with AT commonly present with progressive cerebellar ataxia, oculocutaneous telangiectasia and clinical manifestations of immune deficiency [30, 33, 36]. It is caused by biallelic mutations in the ataxia-telangiectasia mutated gene (ATM), responsible for DNA repair and located on chromosome 11q22.3-23.1 [30, 33]. ATM is involved in many cellular functions, including cell cycle checkpoint control, apoptosis, DNA damage response (DDR), and more recently, oxidative stress and mitochondrial metabolism. The recognized clinical and biologic heterogeneity in AT is thought to be at least in part associated with the type of ATM mutations [33, 46].

Ataxia telangiectasia is a classic example of a genetic defect that affects immune function and can directly add to oncogenesis [30]. About two-thirds of patients with AT suffer from immune system abnormalities, such as reduced T and B cells and low levels of one or more immunoglobulin classes [47]. In AT, the machinery for double-stranded DNA break repair is affected. This machinery is critical for 'variable diversity and joining' or V(D)J recombination of antigen receptors and thereby the development of functional B and T-cells, but is also involved in repair of DNA damage that could lead to cancer, thus independently predisposing to cancer development as well as affecting immune function.[30]

The lifetime risk of patients with AT to develop cancers is approximately 25%. The most common cancers that occur in patients less than 20 years of age are lymphomas [33, 47-49]. In earlier studies, the most frequent lymphoid malignancy, was T-cell acute lymphoblastic leukemia/lymphoma, more recently, B-NHL is reported to be most frequent [4, 8, 48-50].

The largest study of cancer in patients with AT was a cohort of French patients consisting of 69 patients with cancers identified among 279 patients with AT (24.5%). The most frequent cancer was NHL in 38 patients, of whom 26 had B-NHL. Epstein-Barr virus was associated with 50% of the NHL. The subtypes of B-NHL were not specified in the study. There was a male predominance in patients with NHL, and the median age at NHL diagnosis was 9.7 years. Twenty eight of 38 patients with NHL (73%) were below 15 years of age at time of diagnosis [33].

5.1.2. Nijmegen Breakage Syndrome (NBS)

The defective NBS gene (NBS1, nibrin, or p95) is thought to be a component of the same protein complex or pathway as the AT gene, with each gene possibly coding for proteins contributing to a multi subunit protein involved in correcting radiation induced chromosomal aberrations [5]. The European Society for Immune Deficiencies (EISD) analyzed 149 patients with Nijmegen breakage syndrome (NBS). These patients were clinically heterogeneous, with variable immune deficiencies, ranging from negligible to severe immune dysfunction. Humoral deficiencies predisposed NBS patients to recurrent/chronic respiratory tract infections and worsened long-term prognosis. Eighty malignancies were diagnosed in 63 patients (42%), with malignancy being the leading cause of death in this cohort. Most were of lymphoid origin, and the most common was NHL. Survival probabilities at 5, 10, 20 and 30 years of age were 95, 85, 50 and 35%, respectively, and were significantly lower in patients with than without malignancies [34].

5.1.3. Bloom Syndrome (BS)

Patients with BS characteristically suffer from growth deficiency, photosensitive skin changes, immune deficiency, insulin resistance, a greatly increased risk of early onset of cancer and the development of multiple cancers. Loss-of-function mutations of *BLM*, which codes for a RecQ helicase, results in a functional defect of BLM protein and causes chromosome instability, excessive homologous recombination, and a greatly increased number of sister chromatid exchanges that are pathognomonic of the syndrome [51]. Of the 226 malignant neoplasms diagnosed in 145 people in the Bloom Syndrome Registry (1954-2018), 37 were lymphoma, second only to all acute leukemias. Lymphoma subtype was not specified in the registry [52].

5.2. Wiskott-Aldrich Syndrome (WAS)

Individuals with WAS have a spectrum of presentations, including micro-thrombocytopenia, eczema, and immunodeficiency [53]. Wiskott-Aldrich syndrome is caused by mutations in the WAS gene, which encodes the WAS protein, a key regulator of cell signaling and cytoskeleton reorganization in hematopoietic stem cells. Both T- and B-lymphocyte functions are affected [53, 54]. Susceptibility to cancer development may also be related to alterations of immune surveillance including defective natural killer cell function [1, 54, 55]. The risk for malignancy in patients with WAS gene defects is approximately 100-fold greater than unaffected healthy individuals of similar age, affecting 13–23% of all patients. Malignancies are more common in adolescence and young adulthood. Up to 90% of the malignancies are hematological, with NHL being the most common and DLBCL being the most frequent subtype. Burkitt lymphoma has also been reported [3, 4, 54-62].

5.3. Common Variable Immunodeficiency (CVID)

Impairments in B-cell maturation, such as in the heterogeneous group of common variable immunodeficiency (CVID), primarily yield to humoral immunodeficiencies that are associated with a congenital disorder of B-cell differentiation, B-cell receptor editing, and altered B-cell lifecycle [1]. In CVID, the increased risk for lymphoma is likely multifactorial, including impaired control of EBV-driven lymphoproliferation and genetic instability of lymphocytes due to sustained activation and proliferation during chronic infections [1, 26, 28, 63].

5.4. X-linked Lymphoproliferative Disease Type 1 (XLP1)

X-linked lymphoproliferative disease type 1(XLP1) is characterized by a dysregulated immune response. The mutated gene SH2D1A encodes the signaling lymphocyte activation molecule associated protein, an adaptor protein that has important roles in regulating intracellular signaling [64]. X-linked lymphoproliferative disease type 1 is associated with the development of lymphoma [4, 16]. B- Non Hodgkin lymphoma is the most common type occurring in 25% of patients with XLP1, and is frequently of BL subtype. Affected patients are at risk of developing subsequent B-NHL. Most are extranodal in location and commonly involve the ileocecal region [4, 16, 65-72].

5.5. Other PIDs Associated with Burkitt Lymphoma

One of the major causes of morbidity and mortality in patients with autoimmune lymphoproliferative syndrome (ALPS) is the development of lymphoma. In a study from the National Institutes of Health (NIH) in patients with ALPS, 2 of 7 patients who developed lymphoma had BL, one was EBV positive. The diagnosis of BL was made at age 17 and 50 years. Both were long term survivors at the time of publication. One received cyclophosphamide, vincristine and prednisone (COP), while treatment details were not described in the other [73].

Other less frequent PIDs associated with B-NHL is in patients with Di George syndrome, 4 patients were described with DLBCL and none with BL [74-77].

6. Treatment Considerations

The management of patients with PID-BL remains a challenging, yet fortunately, rare, effort. The rarity of these conditions is partly responsible for the difficult and slow pace of scientific advancement in this field [5].

Overall, individuals with PIDs-associated lymphomas are at high risk of suffering from more severe treatment-related toxicities. Each PID deserves special treatment considerations based on the unique risk factors caused by the underlying defect and pathophysiology. The most compelling example is treatment planning and preemptive decision making when B-NHL is diagnosed in an individual with a chromosome instability syndrome. These are associated with severe chemotherapy-related toxicities, particularly severe myelosuppression and sepsis [33, 34, 36, 39].

6.1. Index of Suspicion of PIDs in Newly Diagnosed B-NHL

With broader awareness of the different PIDs clinical phenotypes, along with the availability of reliable diagnostic tools, the incidence of these disorders might be much higher than reported. It is possible that there are more undiagnosed cases of PIDs among pediatric patients with lymphoid malignancies [54, 78]. In a study by Seidemann et al., 3 of 19 patients with PIDs and NHL, the diagnosis of lymphoma was made prior to PIDs. In these cases, several findings prompted further immunological investigations and diagnosis of specific immunodeficiency syndromes. These were, very young age (below 3 years at the time of lymphoma diagnosis), or very limited tolerance of chemotherapy with severe mucositis and recurrent sepsis. These findings and further investigations led to the diagnosis and characterization of immune deficiency while patients were receiving chemotherapy and resulted in making the individual diagnoses of AT or NBS in 3 patients [20].

6.2. Chemotherapy

A recent large multicenter study in pediatric patients with NHL identified 213 lymphomas in patients with predisposing conditions, including 32 patients with AT and 26 with NBS. Some of these patients were treated according to institutional treatment guidelines for children with PIDs/chromosomal breakage syndromes. Of the 213 patients, 174 (82%) were treated according to cooperative group protocols. The remaining 39 patients (18%) received CHOP ± rituximab (cyclophosphamide, hydroxy doxorubicin, vincristine and prednisolone ± rituximab), COP ± rituximab (cyclophosphamide, vincristine and prednisolone ± rituximab), rituximab only, or miscellaneous treatments. Compared to immunocompetent patients, there was an inferior survival rate. For the 151 patients with a known cancer risk, 5-year event-free survival (EFS) and overall survival (OS) rates were 40% ± 4% and 51% ± 4%, respectively. Five-year cumulative incidences of progression/relapse and treatment-related death as a first event were 22% ± 4% and 24% ± 4%, respectively. There was a large proportion of therapy-related deaths compared to immunocompetent patients with NHL. The survey asked for information about dose reductions, withholding of components of chemotherapy or single drugs, and individualized therapy approaches. Unfortunately, these were not uniformly reported in all patients making it impossible to assess whether modifications of therapy influenced therapy-related toxicity and mortality, response and outcome [8].

Treatment refractoriness has also been reported in a study from a large center in Italy, only half of the patients (13 of 25) with hematologic malignancies survived. The outcome of 16 patients who had NHL in this study was particularly poor with lymphoma as the major cause of death. Among these, 3 had suboptimal responses leading to progression and 6 patients relapsed [27].

6.3. Special Treatment Considerations in PIDs Associated BL

6.3.1. Chromosome Instability Syndromes

Patients with PIDs who develop lymphomas associated with chromosome breakage syndromes, such as AT, NBS and BS, poorly tolerate full dose chemotherapy and are at high risk of severe and life-threatening complications of prolonged severe myelosuppression, sepsis and in some, neurologic and pulmonary toxicity. Therefore, treatment reductions are often necessary [33, 34, 36, 39, 40, 51, 52, 79]. In the majority of patients, drug doses are reduced especially at the beginning of treatment and escalated based on the individual response and toxicity profile [36]. Despite this, few specific treatment modifications guidelines exist [8, 52]. Sandlund et al., provided several preventive recommendations for the treatment of NHL in patients with AT. These included 25% dose reduction of daunorubicin and etoposide, administration of mesna with all cyclophosphamide and ifosfamide doses to decrease risk of late onset hemorrhagic cystitis, and limiting the use of vinca alkaloid. In addition to prompt and early intervention with broad spectrum antibiotics when infection is suspected, they recommended particular attention to avoid the concomitant use of nephrotoxic drugs, to optimize methotrexate clearance [39].

6.3.2. Ataxia Telangiectasia and Nijmegen Breakage Syndrome

In the largest cohort of 69 patients with AT who developed cancer, overall survival was shorter in patients with AT who developed cancer compared with those who did not (15 *vs* 24 years, respectively; P .001). Survival was improved in patients who achieved a major response to treatment (3.46 *vs* 0.87 years for major *vs* minor responses, respectively; P .011) [33].

One of the most informative studies addressing treatment modifications and therapy-related toxicities was by Bienemann et al. In their study all 20 pediatric patients with AT or NBS who developed B-NHL were treated according to NHL-BFM therapy. Five of 20 patients received all courses at the scheduled dose without any modifications. Four patients received one or two courses at full dose and the remaining courses at a reduced dose. The other 11 patients received modified treatment with significant dose reduction from the start to the end of therapy. Dose reductions included methotrexate dose reduction to 1 g/m^2 instead of 5 g/m^2. Some doses were completely omitted. Drug doses were subsequently increased during the following courses according to individual tolerance. One patient was switched to monoclonal antibody therapy alone after two chemotherapy courses because of severe toxicity. In the entire cohort of 37 patients with lymphoid malignancies, grade 3 or 4 toxicities occurred in all patients, the most common were mucositis, sepsis and enterocolitis [36].

In the same study, patients with NBS experienced more toxicity. There was a clear reduction of these side effects in patients who had dose reduction. All patients who received full dose chemotherapy developed severe toxicity after more than 50% of the courses, while only two of the 16 patients treated with reduced dose schedules developed severe toxicity after more than 50% of the courses. Six of these 16 patients developed no severe toxicities at all. In one patient, chemotherapy had to be aborted because of life-threatening toxicity and another died of sepsis after a dose-reduced chemotherapy course. Of 20 patients with either AT or NBS and B-NHL, 11 survived. Of the nine patients who died: two died of lymphoma progression, and two of a progressive second or third malignancy. One patient died of therapy-associated toxicity after the fourth course of chemotherapy, three patients died of an infection as a result of PIDs and one of respiratory failure due to chronic lung disease [36].

Rituximab was administered to 4 of the 20 patients in the study by Bienemann et al., three of them were long term survivors. One of the survivors did not tolerate chemotherapy and was switched to monotherapy with rituximab and remained in complete remission 4 years after diagnosis. Two additional patients were successfully treated with rituximab, one who had a second B-NHL was treated with rituximab monotherapy. The other was treated for early relapse with rituximab and two courses of CHOP [36].

In another institutional study of 5 patients with AT who developed B-NHL, (one had BL), only one survived. Causes of death were induction failure, relapse, sepsis and delayed onset lung disease. The authors suggested that the occurrence of induction failure in one of the 5 patients raises suspicion that malignancies occurring in children with AT may be more resistant to standard therapy, and hypothesized that this could be secondary to unidentified high-risk biological characteristics Another hypothesis was possible decreased chemotherapy-induced apoptotic signaling in the transformed cells, due to lack of ATM, resulting in inherent, biologically-resistant disease' [39].

6.3.3. Nijmegen Breakage Syndrome

Two studies offered specific treatment modification and toxicity data in NBS. One was the study by Bienemann et al. In another study of 17 patients with NBS with lymphoid malignancies, 8 developed 13 B-NHL. Three patients experienced two or more B-NHL. There were two BL and 11 DLBCL (Table 2). The outcome was poor with only 6 of 17 patients surviving. All patients with B-NHL and available chemotherapy data received LMB-based chemotherapy for at least one B-NHL. One patient received R-CHOP for the second of 3 lymphomas. Among 17 patients, 7 received more and 10 received less than 80% of protocol-specified drug doses. Response to chemotherapy was similar in both groups. Despite this, 11 of 17 patients died, two from treatment-related complications and the others from disease relapse/progression. Time from diagnosis to death from lymphoma ranged from 3 months to 3.5 years (median: 1.1 year). There were no differences in the number of grade 3 and 4 toxicities in patients receiving less or more than 80% of drug doses, and the two treatment-related deaths were in patients who received less than 80% of drug doses during their last course of chemotherapy. Six of seven patients who received over 80% of drug doses were alive, while most patients who received less than 80% died either from lymphoma or other complications [80].

6.3.4. Bloom Syndrome

Chemotherapy dose reduction is often necessary when initial chemotherapy is given to patients with BS. Individuals with BS have usually tolerated doses at or below 50% of the standard chemotherapy dosage. However, full dose may be appropriate for some components of immunochemotherapeutic regimen such as corticosteroids and rituximab. Absence of information about the ideal doses makes such treatment decisions particularly challenging in clinical practice [40, 52]. A 5-year-old boy with abdominal BL who was treated with LMB protocol, tolerated chemotherapy poorly. After an initial response, the tumor progressed and he died of lymphoma 14 months after initial diagnosis [40]. Another 11-year-old with Bloom syndrome and BL, had minimal therapeutic response and significant dose-limiting toxicity with standard chemotherapy, but subsequently responded to rituximab combined with mild chemotherapy (vincristine and prednisone) and was alive in remission, 4 years after end of therapy [79].

6.3.5. Wiscott Aldrich Syndrome

Individuals with WAS-associated lymphoma described in the literature were treated according to various regimens that included surgery and or radiotherapy in earlier reports. More recently they were treated with chemotherapy, with or without immunotherapy [56-60]. Despite lack of guidelines on the best treatment or its modification, the presence of thrombocytopenia and primary immunodeficiency justifies reduction of chemotherapy doses to reduce the risk of life-threatening treatment related complications [56, 58, 60].

Burkitt lymphoma has been rarely reported in patients with WAS. A 12-year-old patient with an ileocecal mass was found to have EBV positive BL. He was subsequently diagnosed with WAS. The patient was treated with four courses of cyclophosphamide, vincristine, and prednisone (COP) with the addition of rituximab during the first two courses. He tolerated chemotherapy well and complete remission was achieved. The authors did not describe the details of chemotherapy intensity or duration of remission [41]. Most cases of NHL in patients with WAS are of the mature B-subtype, mostly DLBCL. Because of the paucity of published treatment and outcome data in BL associated with WAS, we summarize here the limited data available in WAS-associated DLBCL, which could provide insights on the patients' treatment and outcome. A review by Senapati et al., included 23 cases of NHL, 12 with DLBCL and only the patient described by Pasic et al., had BL. [41, 81] In the remaining cases, NHL subtype was not specified. There were individual case reports of 5 males (age 9-16) with DLBCL, one of which was EBV positive. Three patients survived 0.5, 3, and 9 years from diagnosis, while the other 2 died, one of sepsis and the other from surgical complications. As expected they were treated with various regimens and intensities [60, 81-84]. The 3 survivors in the modern era received multiagent chemotherapy regimens used in mature B cell lymphoma and included: LNH97 with 75% dose reduction, localized B-NHL regimen that was escalated to cisplatin-based regimen for progression, and one received 4 cycles of R-CHOP [60, 81, 82].

6.3.6. X-linked Lymphoproliferative Disease Type 1

Patients with XLP1 are at particularly high risk of developing second lymphomas and importantly they are even at higher risk of, often fatal, HLH driven fulminant EBV (fEBV). Therefore, the diagnosis of XLP1 should prompt consideration of allogeneic SCT from an unaffected donor. If successful, this is expected to reduce the risk of fEBV and of a second or third lymphoma. Few publications describe the outcome of these transplanted patients, and long term follow up is unavailable [16, 67]. It is important to identify other affected males and female carriers in the family; the latter can then be offered prenatal diagnosis or arrangements made to screen male infants at birth [16].

6.4. Treatment Modalities Other Than Chemotherapy

6.4.1. Targeted Immunotherapy

As already proven in adults, rituximab in combination with chemotherapy has been proven to improve outcome in children and adults with high risk BL and DLBCL, without major added toxicities [13, 85-87]. On the other hand, the role of rituximab in allowing chemotherapy reduction without impairing lymphoma outcome has not been prospectively studied in IC patients with B-NHL.

Similarly, there are no prospective studies, in patients with PIDs, of the impact of rituximab in allowing chemotherapy reduction without reducing lymphoma-free survival. Successful use of rituximab in combination with chemotherapy in PIDs-associated lymphoma has been reported in one case series and an individual case report [36, 79]. These cases provide some evidence of the efficacy of rituximab in allowing treatment reduction for B-NHL in patients with PIDs, but its impact on event free survival is unknown.

Second generation CD-20 directed antibodies have not replaced rituximab in first line therapy in DLBCL [88], and their use has not been reported in B-NHL associated with PIDs. More recently, bispecific CD20 X CD3 antibodies have entered clinical trials in B-NHL [89]. Since these antibodies engage T-cell to induce tumor cytotoxicity, they are not likely to play a future role in the treatment of B-NHL occurring in combined or T cell immune deficiency disorders.

The concept of manufacturing autologous chimeric antigen receptor T cell (CART-T) from patients with PIDs face similar challenges. Autologous CAR-T directed against CD19 have shown efficacy in relapsed refractory (r/r) B-ALL and r/r DLBCL, and are FDA approved for these indications [90-94]. However the experience in patients with R/R BL is limited to case reports [95, 96].

6.4.2. EBV Specific Cytotoxic T cells

Limited experience exists about the use of EBV specific cytotoxic T cells in B-NHL in immunocompetent patients. Some responses have been observed to the administration to LMP– cytotoxic T lymphocytes (CTLs) to heavily pretreated relapsed refractory DLBCL in adults [97]. Currently, the concept of sensitizing BL to EBV-CTLs is being explored [98]. The potential therapeutic value of this therapy in EBV-positive PIDs-associated B-NHL has not been studied.

6.4.3. Allogeneic Hematopoietic Stem Cell Transplantation (HSCT)

Allogeneic hematopoietic stem cell transplantation (HSCT), a standard treatment in patients with SCID and WAS, has the advantage of immune reconstitution, and therefore the reduction of the risk of PIDs-associated lymphoma. However, there is some evidence that performing HSCT after developing a hematologic malignancy may be insufficient in the control of these tumors, as lymphoma relapses have been reported after HSCT [27]. On the other hand, in patients with XLP1, lymphoma is often the initial presentation of the underlying immune disorder. In these patients HSCT is an important treatment option to prevent further lymphomas and fatal HLH driven by fEBV infection [16, 66]. The anti-tumor efficacy of T cell reconstitution in the allogeneic HSCT setting is illustrated by a case described by Mustillo et al., This was a 7 month- old with X linked SCIDS, who developed DLBCL of the orbit. Initial chemotherapy and rituximab resulted only in partial response, with 50% decrease in the size of the tumor prior to HSCT. Even after fludarabine conditioning for HSCT, the tumor showed no response and progressed by 100 days posttransplant. Complete resolution occurred only after 100% donor chimerism was achieved and there was evidence of functional donor T-lymphocytes by 180 days after HSCT. The infant died 3 months later of an unrelated surgical complication. Interestingly, the tumor was EBV-negative, therefore illustrating that the cancer predilection associated with immunodeficient hosts may not be a specific immune defect in the recognition of viral specific antigens, but rather a defect in immune surveillance necessary for elimination of cells with abnormalities in proliferation, function and/or apoptosis. Another instructive point was the strong temporal association between the recovery of donor T-cell function and complete resolution of the lymphoma [45].

Table 4. Clinical practice gaps and areas of future investigation

Clinical question			
Gap	Barrier	Potential practice change	Clinical implications
Undiagnosed cases of PIDs at initial diagnosis of lymphoma	Small number of patients (diluted experience)	High index of suspicion of a potentially undiagnosed PID	Preemptive modification of chemotherapy doses based on the suspected type of PID Guide treatment decisions and minimize treatment complications
Areas of future investigation			
Knowledge gap	Research question	Area of investigation	Purpose
Epidemiologic differences	Much smaller number of BL compared to DLBCL in patients with PIDs compared to IC children	Genomic studies of potential differences between BL and DLBCL occurring in IC compared to patients with PIDs	Better understanding of pathobiology that could provide clues for therapeutic strategies and targeted therapy
Therapeutic questions	Role of rituximab Chemotherapy modifications due to increased risk of therapy-related toxicity and overall poor outcome	Observational studies: Build strata for patients with PIDs in lymphoma clinical trials Cancer registries/PIDs registries: Incorporate cancer treatment details, toxicities and outcome in data bases	Build body of evidence to define the impact of rituximab in allowing chemotherapy reduction without reducing lymphoma-free survival Develop consensus guidelines for the incorporation of rituximab in treatment regimens and for chemotherapy modifications

BL: Burkitt lymphoma; DLBCL: diffuse large B cell lymphoma; PIDs; primary immune deficiency disorders; IC: immunocompetent.

With the exception of SCID and WAS, experience with HSCT in patients with PIDs predisposed to NHL, particularly DNA repair disorders, is limited. HSCT has been performed with some success in patients with NBS and was proposed for patients in first remission of lymphoma, given its potential to replace the tissue that is prone to future primary and secondary malignant transformation [34, 99]. Recently, a large retrospective multicenter study was conducted to evaluate the feasibility and outcome of HSCT in DNA repair defects; included in this cohort of 87 patients were patients with NBS and AT. The OS of this group was 69%. Deaths mostly occurred early after SCT and significantly more frequently in patients who had been treated with myeloablative conditioning compared with those who received reduced-intensity regimens. Patients with AT had the poorest outcome with only 25% survival, leading to the conclusion that HSCT should not be routinely recommended in patients with AT. No secondary malignancies were observed in this cohort during the relatively short median follow-up period of 35 months [1, 100].

7. Unique Long Term Risks

7.1. Malignancies

Second and third malignancies are the ultimate challenge in patients with PIDs. In the study by Attarbaschi et al., of 151 patients with conditions predisposing to malignancy, the 10-year incidence of second malignancy was 24% ± 5% and 7-year OS of the 21 patients with a second malignancy was 41% ± 11% [8]. Similarly, in a study of patients with AT and NBS who developed NHL, 10 of 20 patients developed second malignancies (26%) with a median latency of 3- 5 years after diagnosis of the first lymphoid malignancy. Six of these subsequent malignancies were NHL. Three patients were alive after successful treatment of a second lymphoid malignancy [36]. This risk of a second malignancy is in line with similar studies [27, 52].

7.2. Chronic Lung Disease

Chronic lung disease is a serious complication and a significant cause of early mortality of a number of PIDs, such as AT and BS [51, 52, 101, 102]. It is not known if chemotherapy administration and or its related infectious complications accelerate this process in some patients, as in the patient described at the start of this chapter (case-1). Bienemann et al., described a child who was treated for a second B-NHL with one course of standard BFM therapy reduced at 50%. Despite achieving remission, she died 8 months later of chronic lung disease [36]. In another report, a 19-year-old with AT who was successfully treated for DLBCL with LMB-89 regimen expired 3 years from diagnosis due to pneumonitis [39].

Conclusion and Future Perspectives

Primary immune deficiency disorders are one of the strongest known risk factors for the development of BL and other subtypes of NHL. Despite this, encounter of these cases in clinical practice is a rare event. High index of suspicion of a potentially undiagnosed PIDs when a new diagnosis of BL is made can guide treatment decisions and minimize treatment complications by preemptive modification of chemotherapy doses based on the suspected type of PIDs. Despite excellent outcome and advances in the study of IC-BL in immunocompetent patients, management of BL in patients with PIDs remains difficult, because of their small numbers, increased risk of therapy-related toxicity and overall poor outcome. Because of these unique features, these patients are less studied as they are often excluded from clinical trials. Despite the promise of immunotherapy, its increasing use alone or in addition to chemotherapy to treat B-NHL in patients with PIDs is limited to individual case reports and case series. There is a great need to develop new therapeutic approaches in this group. Most likely, treatment plans need to be individualized in the context of PIDs specific risk of complications. Prospective studies may not be feasible in these rare diseases, but observational studies in collaboration with registries of patients with PIDs on specific details of cancer treatment including chemotherapy intensity and the inclusion of immunotherapy, can contribute to the knowledge of treatment outcome, determine the best treatment approaches, and future development of PIDs associated B-NHL specific treatment guidelines, with emphasis on the potential role of immunotherapy in allowing chemotherapy reduction and reducing treatment related morbidity and mortality (Table 4).

ACKNOWLEDGMENTS

The authors wish to thank Dr. Denis Miller for reviewing this chapter.

REFERENCES

[1] Hauck, F., R. Voss, C. Urban, and M. G. Seidel. 2018. "Intrinsic and extrinsic causes of malignancies in patients with primary immunodeficiency disorders." *J Allergy Clin Immunol* 141 (1):59-68 e4. doi: 10.1016/j.jaci.2017.06.009.

[2] Mueller, B. U., and P. A. Pizzo. 1995. "Cancer in children with primary or secondary immunodeficiencies." *J Pediatr* 126 (1):1-10.

[3] Tran, H., J. Nourse, S. Hall, M. Green, L. Griffiths, and M. K. Gandhi. 2008. "Immunodeficiency-associated lymphomas." *Blood Rev* 22 (5):261-81. doi: 10.1016/j.blre.2008.03.009.

[4] Duan, L., and E. Grunebaum. 2018. "Hematological Malignancies Associated With Primary Immunodeficiency Disorders." *Clin Immunol* 194:46-59. doi: 10.1016/j.clim.2018.06.011.

[5] Shapiro, R. S. 2011. "Malignancies in the setting of primary immunodeficiency: Implications for hematologists/oncologists." *Am J Hematol* 86 (1):48-55. doi: 10.1002/ajh.21903.

[6] Gross, Thomas G., and Shiramizu, Bruce. 2007. "Lymphoproliferative disorders related to immunodeficiencies." In: *Pediatric Lymphomas*, 233–58.

[7] Worch, J., M. Rohde, and B. Burkhardt. 2013. "Mature B-cell lymphoma and leukemia in children and adolescents-review of standard chemotherapy regimen and perspectives." *Pediatr Hematol Oncol* 30 (6):465-83. doi: 10.3109/08880018.2013.783891.

[8] Attarbaschi, A., E. Carraro, O. Abla, S. Barzilai-Birenboim, S. Bomken, L. Brugieres, E. Bubanska, B. Burkhardt, A. K. Chiang, M. Csoka, A. Fedorova, J. Jazbec, E. Kabickova, Z. Krenova, J. Lazic, J. Loeffen, G. Mann, F. Niggli, N. Miakova, T. Osumi, L. Ronceray, A. Uyttebroeck, D. Williams, W. Woessmann, G. Wrobel, M. Pillon, Lymphoma European Intergroup for Childhood Non-Hodgkin, and Group the International Berlin-Frankfur t-Munster Study. 2016. "Non-Hodgkin lymphoma and pre-existing conditions: spectrum, clinical characteristics and outcome in 213 children and adolescents." *Haematologica* 101 (12):1581-1591. doi: 10.3324/haematol.2016.147116.

[9] Meinhardt, A., B. Burkhardt, M. Zimmermann, A. Borkhardt, U. Kontny, T. Klingebiel, F. Berthold, G. Janka-Schaub, C. Klein, E. Kabickova, W. Klapper, A. Attarbaschi, M. Schrappe, A. Reiter, and group Berlin-Frankfurt-Munster. 2010. "Phase II window study on rituximab in newly diagnosed pediatric mature B-cell non-Hodgkin's lymphoma and Burkitt leukemia." *J Clin Oncol* 28 (19):3115-21. doi: 10.1200/JCO.2009.26.6791.

[10] Cairo, M. S., R. Sposto, M. Gerrard, A. Auperin, S. C. Goldman, L. Harrison, R. Pinkerton, M. Raphael, K. McCarthy, S. L. Perkins, and C. Patte. 2012. "Advanced stage, increased lactate dehydrogenase, and primary site, but not adolescent age (>/=15 years), are associated with an increased risk of treatment failure in children and adolescents with mature B-cell non-Hodgkin's lymphoma: results of the FAB LMB 96 study." *J Clin Oncol* 30 (4):387-93. doi: 10.1200/JCO.2010.33.3369.

[11] Cairo, M. S., M. Gerrard, R. Sposto, A. Auperin, C. R. Pinkerton, J. Michon, C. Weston, S. L. Perkins, M. Raphael, K. McCarthy, C. Patte, and FAB LMB International Study Committee. 2007. "Results of a randomized international study of high-risk central nervous system B non-Hodgkin lymphoma and B acute lymphoblastic leukemia in children and adolescents." *Blood* 109 (7):2736-43. doi: 10.1182/blood-2006-07-036665.

[12] Patte, C., A. Auperin, M. Gerrard, J. Michon, R. Pinkerton, R. Sposto, C. Weston, M. Raphael, S. L. Perkins, K. McCarthy, M. S. Cairo, and Fab Lmb International Study Committee. 2007. "Results of the randomized international FAB/LMB96 trial for intermediate risk B-cell non-Hodgkin lymphoma in children and adolescents: it is possible to reduce treatment for the early responding patients." *Blood* 109 (7):2773-80. doi: 10.1182/blood-2006-07-036673.

[13] Minard-Colin, V., Auperin, A., Pillon, M., Burke, G. A. A., Barkauskas, D. A., Wheatley, K., Delgado, R. F., Alexander, S., Uyttebroeck, A., Bollard, C. M., Zsiros, J., Csoka, M., Kazanowska, B., Chiang, A. K., Miles, R. R., Wotherspoon, A., Adamson, P. C., Vassal, G., Patte, C., Gross, T. G., European Intergroup for Childhood Non-Hodgkin, Lymphoma, and Children's Oncology, Group. 2020. "Rituximab for High-Risk, Mature B-Cell Non-Hodgkin's Lymphoma in Children." *N Engl J Med* 382 (23):2207-2219. doi: 10.1056/NEJMoa1915315.

[14] Woessmann, W., K. Seidemann, G. Mann, M. Zimmermann, B. Burkhardt, I. Oschlies, W. D. Ludwig, T. Klingebiel, N. Graf, B. Gruhn, H. Juergens, F. Niggli, R. Parwaresch, H. Gadner, H. Riehm, M. Schrappe, A. Reiter, and B. F. M. Group. 2005. "The impact of the methotrexate administration schedule and dose in the treatment of children and adolescents with B-cell neoplasms: a report of the BFM Group Study NHL-BFM95." *Blood* 105 (3):948-58. doi: 10.1182/blood-2004-03-0973.

[15] Ours, C., A. Cunningham, Z. Afify. 2018. "Unique presentations of ataxia-telangiectasia in two brothers." *Pediatric Blood and Cancer;* 65: S21,0.13.

[16] Iglesias Cardenas, F., A M. Agarwal, J. Vagher, L. Maese, M. Fluchel, Z. Afify. 2021. Two Clonally Distinct B-Cell Lymphomas Reveal the Diagnosis of XLP1 in a Male Child and His Asymptomatic Male Relatives: Case Report and Review of the Literature. *J Pediatr Hematol Oncol*. Epub ahead of print. DOI: 10.1097/MPH.0000000000002049.

[17] Sullivan, K. E., J. M. Puck, L. D. Notarangelo, R. Fuleihan, T. Caulder, C. Wang, M. Boyle, and C. Cunningham-Rundles. 2014. "USIDNET: a strategy to build a community of clinical immunologists." *J Clin Immunol* 34 (4):428-35. doi: 10.1007/s10875-014-0028-1.

[18] Filipovich, A. H., K. J. Heinitz, L. L. Robison, and G. Frizzera. 1987. "The Immunodeficiency Cancer Registry. A research resource." *Am J Pediatr Hematol Oncol* 9 (2):183-4. doi: 10.1097/00043426-198722000-00017.

[19] Filipovich, A. H., A. Mathur, D. Kamat, and R. S. Shapiro. 1992. "Primary immunodeficiencies: genetic risk factors for lymphoma." *Cancer Res* 52 (19 Suppl):5465s-5467s.

[20] Seidemann, K., M. Tiemann, G. Henze, A. Sauerbrey, S. Muller, and A. Reiter. 1999. "Therapy for non-Hodgkin lymphoma in children with primary immunodeficiency: analysis of 19 patients from the BFM trials." *Med Pediatr Oncol* 33 (6):536-44. doi: 10.1002/(sici)1096-911x(199912)33:6<536::aid-mpo3>3.0.co;2-z.

[21] Hayward, A. R., J. Levy, F. Facchetti, L. Notarangelo, H. D. Ochs, A. Etzioni, J. Y. Bonnefoy, M. Cosyns, and A. Weinberg. 1997. "Cholangiopathy and tumors of the pancreas, liver, and biliary tree in boys with X-linked immunodeficiency with hyper-IgM." *J Immunol* 158 (2):977-83.

[22] Kersey, J. H., R. S. Shapiro, and A. H. Filipovich. 1988. "Relationship of immunodeficiency to lymphoid malignancy." *Pediatr Infect Dis J* 7 (5 Suppl):S10-2.

[23] Kersey, J. H., B. D. Spector, and R. A. Good. 1974. "Cancer in children with primary immunodeficiency diseases." *J Pediatr* 84 (2):263-4. doi: 10.1016/s0022-3476(74)80619-0.

[24] Mellemkjaer, L., L. Hammarstrom, V. Andersen, J. Yuen, C. Heilmann, T. Barington, J. Bjorkander, and J. H. Olsen. 2002. "Cancer risk among patients with IgA deficiency or common variable immunodeficiency and their relatives: a combined Danish and Swedish study." *Clin Exp Immunol* 130 (3):495-500. doi: 10.1046/j.1365-2249.2002.02004.x.

[25] Robison, L. L., V. Stoker, G. Frizzera, K. Heinitz, A. T. Meadows, and A. H. Filipovich. 1987. "Hodgkin's disease in pediatric patients with naturally occurring immunodeficiency." *Am J Pediatr Hematol Oncol* 9 (2):189-92. doi: 10.1097/00043426-198722000-00019.

[26] Vajdic, C. M., L. Mao, M. T. van Leeuwen, P. Kirkpatrick, A. E. Grulich, and S. Riminton. 2010. "Are antibody deficiency disorders associated with a narrower range of cancers than other forms of immunodeficiency?" *Blood* 116 (8):1228-34. doi: 10.1182/blood-2010-03-272351.

[27] Maffeis, M., L. D. Notarangelo, R. F. Schumacher, E. Soncini, A. Soresina, A. Lanfranchi, and F. Porta. 2019. "Primary Immunodeficiencies and Oncological Risk: The Experience of the Children's Hospital of Brescia." *Front Pediatr* 7:232. doi: 10.3389/fped.2019.00232.

[28] Gathmann, B., N. Mahlaoui, Ceredih, L. Gerard, E. Oksenhendler, K. Warnatz, I. Schulze, G. Kindle, T. W. Kuijpers, W. I. D. Dutch, R. T. van Beem, D. Guzman, S. Workman, P. Soler-Palacin, J. De Gracia, T. Witte, R. E. Schmidt, J. Litzman, E. Hlavackova, V. Thon, M. Borte, S. Borte, D. Kumararatne, C. Feighery, H. Longhurst, M. Helbert, A. Szaflarska, A. Sediva, B. H. Belohradsky, A. Jones, U. Baumann, I. Meyts, N. Kutukculer, P. Wagstrom, N. M. Galal, J. Roesler, E. Farmaki, N. Zinovieva, P. Ciznar, E. Papadopoulou-Alataki, K. Bienemann, S. Velbri, Z. Panahloo, B. Grimbacher, and Party European Society for Immunodeficiencies Registry Working. 2014. "Clinical picture and treatment of 2212 patients with common variable immunodeficiency." *J Allergy Clin Immunol* 134 (1):116-26. doi: 10.1016/j.jaci.2013.12.1077.

[29] Arico, M., L. Mussolin, E. Carraro, S. Buffardi, N. Santoro, P. D'Angelo, A. Lombardi, P. Pierani, E. Giraldi, R. Mura, A. Sala, A. Garaventa, A. Tondo, M. Piglione, L. Lo Nigro, S. Cesaro, K. Perruccio, A. Rosolen, G. Basso, M. Pillon, and N. HL-Committee of the Italian Association of Pediatric Hematology Oncology. 2015. "Non-Hodgkin lymphoma in children with an associated inherited condition: A retrospective analysis of the Associazione Italiana Ematologia Oncologia Pediatrica (AIEOP)." *Pediatr Blood Cancer* 62 (10):1782-9. doi: 10.1002/pbc.25565.

[30] Verhoeven, D., A. J. Stoppelenburg, F. Meyer-Wentrup, and M. Boes. 2018. "Increased risk of hematologic malignancies in primary immunodeficiency disorders: opportunities for immunotherapy." *Clin Immunol* 190:22-31. doi: 10.1016/j.clim.2018.02.007.

[31] Seidemann, K., G. Henze, J. D. Beck, A. Sauerbrey, J. Kuhl, G. Mann, and A. Reiter. 2000. "Non-Hodgkin's lymphoma in pediatric patients with chromosomal breakage syndromes (AT and NBS): experience from the BFM trials." *Ann Oncol* 11 Suppl 1:141-5.

[32] Jonkman-Berk, B. M., J. M. van den Berg, I. J. Ten Berge, R. G. Bredius, G. J. Driessen, V. A. Dalm, J. T. van Dissel, M. van Deuren, P. M. Ellerbroek, M. van der Flier, P. M. van Hagen, J. M. van Montfrans, A. Rutgers, E. H. Scholvinck, E. de Vries, R. T. van Beem, and T. W. Kuijpers. 2015. "Primary immunodeficiencies in the Netherlands: national patient data demonstrate the increased risk of malignancy." *Clin Immunol* 156 (2):154-62. doi: 10.1016/j.clim.2014.10.003.

[33] Suarez, F., N. Mahlaoui, D. Canioni, C. Andriamanga, C. Dubois d'Enghien, N. Brousse, J. P. Jais, A. Fischer, O. Hermine, and D. Stoppa-Lyonnet. 2015. "Incidence, presentation, and prognosis of malignancies in ataxia-telangiectasia: a report from the French national registry of primary immune deficiencies." *J Clin Oncol* 33 (2):202-8. doi: 10.1200/JCO.2014.56.5101.

[34] Wolska-Kusnierz, B., H. Gregorek, K. Chrzanowska, B. Piatosa, B. Pietrucha, E. Heropolitanska-Pliszka, M. Pac, M. Klaudel-Dreszler, L. Kostyuchenko, S. Pasic, L. Marodi, B. H. Belohradsky, P. Ciznar,

A. Shcherbina, S. S. Kilic, U. Baumann, M. G. Seidel, A. R. Gennery, M. Syczewska, B. Mikoluc, K. Kalwak, J. Styczynski, A. Pieczonka, K. Drabko, A. Wakulinska, B. Gathmann, M. H. Albert, U. Skarzynska, E. Bernatowska, on behalf of the Inborn Errors Working Party of the Society for European, Transplantation Marrow, and Deficiencies the European Society for Immune. 2015. "Nijmegen Breakage Syndrome: Clinical and Immunological Features, Long-Term Outcome and Treatment Options - a Retrospective Analysis." *J Clin Immunol* 35 (6):538-49. doi: 10.1007/s10875-015-0186-9.

[35] Mayor, P. C., K. H. Eng, K. L. Singel, S. I. Abrams, K. Odunsi, K. B. Moysich, R. Fuleihan, E. Garabedian, P. Lugar, H. D. Ochs, F. A. Bonilla, R. H. Buckley, K. E. Sullivan, Z. K. Ballas, C. Cunningham-Rundles, and B. H. Segal. 2018. "Cancer in primary immunodeficiency diseases: Cancer incidence in the United States Immune Deficiency Network Registry." *J Allergy Clin Immunol* 141 (3):1028-1035. doi: 10.1016/j.jaci.2017.05.024.

[36] Bienemann, K., B. Burkhardt, S. Modlich, U. Meyer, A. Moricke, K. Bienemann, C. Mauz-Korholz, G. Escherich, M. Zimmermann, D. Korholz, G. Janka-Schaub, M. Schrappe, A. Reiter, and A. Borkhardt. 2011. "Promising therapy results for lymphoid malignancies in children with chromosomal breakage syndromes (*Ataxia teleangiectasia* or Nijmegen-breakage syndrome): a retrospective survey." *Br J Haematol* 155 (4):468-76. doi: 10.1111/j.1365-2141.2011.08863.x.

[37] Egan, Grace, Weitzman, Sheila, and Alexander, Sarah. 2019. "Burkitt Lymphoma and Diffuse Large B-Cell Lymphoma." In *Non-Hodgkin's Lymphoma in Childhood and Adolescence*, 167-183.

[38] Burkhardt, B., M. Zimmermann, I. Oschlies, F. Niggli, G. Mann, R. Parwaresch, H. Riehm, M. Schrappe, A. Reiter, and B. F. M. Group. 2005. "The impact of age and gender on biology, clinical features and treatment outcome of non-Hodgkin lymphoma in childhood and adolescence." *Br J Haematol* 131 (1):39-49. doi: 10.1111/j.1365-2141.2005.05735.x.

[39] Sandlund, J. T., M. M. Hudson, W. Kennedy, M. Onciu, and M. B. Kastan. 2014. "Pilot study of modified LMB-based therapy for children with ataxia-telangiectasia and advanced stage high grade mature B-cell malignancies." *Pediatr Blood Cancer* 61 (2):360-2. doi: 10.1002/pbc.24696.

[40] Fedhila-Ben Ayed, F., W. Douira-Khomsi, S. Rhayem, M. Jelassi, H. Zribi, M. Chaabouni, M. Khemiri, I. Bellagha, and S. Barsaoui. 2016. "Burkitt lymphoma in a child with Bloom syndrome." *Arch Pediatr* 23 (4):382-4. doi: 10.1016/j.arcped.2015.12.004.

[41] Pasic, S., D. Vujic, S. Djuricic, D. Jevtic, and B. Grujic. 2006. "Burkitt lymphoma-induced ileocolic intussusception in Wiskott-Aldrich syndrome." *J Pediatr Hematol Oncol* 28 (1):48-9.

[42] Perkins, A. S., and J. W. Friedberg. 2008. "Burkitt lymphoma in adults." *Hematology Am Soc Hematol Educ Program*: 341-8. doi: 10.1182/asheducation-2008.1.341.

[43] Roschewski, M., K. Dunleavy, J. S. Abramson, B. L. Powell, B. K. Link, P. Patel, P. J. Bierman, D. Jagadeesh, R. T. Mitsuyasu, D. Peace, P. R. Watson, W. T. Hanna, C. Melani, A. N. Lucas, S. M. Steinberg, S. Pittaluga, E. S. Jaffe, J. W. Friedberg, B. S. Kahl, R. F. Little, N. L. Bartlett, M. A. Fanale, A. Noy, and W. H. Wilson. 2020. "Multicenter Study of Risk-Adapted Therapy with Dose-Adjusted EPOCH-R in Adults With Untreated Burkitt Lymphoma." *J Clin Oncol* 38 (22):2519-2529. doi: 10.1200/JCO.20.00303.

[44] Mustillo Salavoura, K., A. Kolialexi, G. Tsangaris, and A. Mavrou. 2008. "Development of cancer in patients with primary immunodeficiencies." *Anticancer Res* 28 (2B):1263-9.

[45] Mustillo, P., R. P. Bajwa, A. M. Termuhlen, K. Nicol, R. Scherzer, R. Jaffe, A. H. Filipovich, and T. G. Gross. 2008. "Tumor immune surveillance defect of X-linked severe combined immunodeficiency is not Epstein-Barr virus specific." *Pediatr Blood Cancer* 51 (5):706-9. doi: 10.1002/pbc.21651.

[46] Staples, E. R., E. M. McDermott, A. Reiman, P. J. Byrd, S. Ritchie, A. M. Taylor, and E. G. Davies. 2008. "Immunodeficiency in ataxia telangiectasia is correlated strongly with the presence of two null

mutations in the ataxia telangiectasia mutated gene." *Clin Exp Immunol* 153 (2):214-20. doi: 10.1111/j.1365-2249.2008.03684.x..

[47] Haas, Oskar A., and Borkhardt, Arndt. 2019. "Genetic Predisposition to Non-Hodgkin Lymphoma." In *Non-Hodgkin's Lymphoma in Childhood and Adolescence*, 97-110.

[48] Sandoval, C., and M. Swift. 1998. "Treatment of lymphoid malignancies in patients with ataxia-telangiectasia." *Med Pediatr Oncol* 31 (6):491-7. doi: 10.1002/(sici)1096-911x(199812) 31:6<491::aid-mpo5>3.0.co;2-b.

[49] Sandoval, C., and M. Swift. 2003. "Hodgkin disease in ataxia-telangiectasia patients with poor outcomes." *Med Pediatr Oncol* 40 (3):162-6. doi: 10.1002/mpo.10251.

[50] Kaneko, H., R. Inoue, Y. Yamada, K. Kasahara, T. Takami, and N. Kondo. 1996. "Ataxia telangiectasia syndrome with B cell lymphoma." *Clin Genet* 49 (6):331-2. doi: 10.1111/j.1399-0004. 1996.tb03803.x.

[51] Cunniff, C., J. A. Bassetti, and N. A. Ellis. 2017. "Bloom's Syndrome: Clinical Spectrum, Molecular Pathogenesis, and Cancer Predisposition." *Mol Syndromol* 8 (1):4-23. doi: 10.1159/ 000452082.

[52] Flanagan, M., and C. M. Cunniff. Bloom Syndrome. 2006 Mar 22 [Updated 2019 Feb 14]. In: Adam M. P., Ardinger H. H., Pagon R. A, et al., editors. *GeneReviews®* [Internet]. Seattle (WA): University of Washington, Seattle; 1993-2021. https://www.ncbi.nlm.nih.gov/ books/NBK1398/?report=reader.

[53] Sullivan, K. E., C. A. Mullen, R. M. Blaese, and J. A. Winkelstein. 1994. "A multiinstitutional survey of the Wiskott-Aldrich syndrome." *J Pediatr* 125 (6 Pt 1):876-85. doi: 10.1016/s0022-3476(05)82002-5.

[54] Ochs, H. D., and A. J. Thrasher. 2006. "The Wiskott-Aldrich syndrome." *J Allergy Clin Immunol* 117 (4):725-38; quiz 739. doi: 10.1016/j.jaci.2006.02.005.

[55] Bosticardo, M., F. Marangoni, A. Aiuti, A. Villa, and M. Grazia Roncarolo. 2009. "Recent advances in understanding the

pathophysiology of Wiskott-Aldrich syndrome." *Blood* 113 (25):6288-95. doi: 10.1182/blood-2008-12-115253.

[56] Koga, Y., H. Takada, A. Suminoe, S. Ohga, and T. Hara. 2014. "Successful treatment of non-Hodgkin's lymphoma using R-CHOP in a patient with Wiskott-Aldrich syndrome followed by a reduced-intensity stem cell transplant." *Pediatr Transplant* 18 (6):E208-11. doi: 10.1111/petr.12297..

[57] Emir, S., E. Vezir, D. Azkur, H. A. Demir, and A. Metin. 2013. "Characteristics of children with non-hodgkin lymphoma associated with primary immune deficiency diseases: descriptions of five patients." *Pediatr Hematol Oncol* 30 (6):544-53. doi: 10.3109/08880018.2013.792893.

[58] Tavil, B., A. Y. Erdem, F. Azik, P. Isik, A. Metin, S. Emir, D. Uckan, and B. Tunc. 2013. "Successful allogeneic hemopoietic stem cell transplantation in a case of Wiskott-Aldrich syndrome and non-Hodgkin lymphoma." *Pediatr Transplant* 17 (6):E146-8. doi: 10.1111/petr.12114.

[59] Yoshimi, A., Y. Kamachi, K. Imai, N. Watanabe, H. Nakadate, T. Kanazawa, S. Ozono, R. Kobayashi, M. Yoshida, C. Kobayashi, A. Hama, H. Muramatsu, Y. Sasahara, M. Jakob, T. Morio, S. Ehl, A. Manabe, C. Niemeyer, and S. Kojima. 2013. "Wiskott-Aldrich syndrome presenting with a clinical picture mimicking juvenile myelomonocytic leukaemia." *Pediatr Blood Cancer* 60 (5):836-41. doi: 10.1002/pbc.24359.

[60] Coccia, P., S. Mastrangelo, A. Ruggiero, M. Scalzone, A. Rosolen, P. Maurizi, and R. Riccardi. 2012. "Treatment of pharyngeal non-Hodgkin lymphoma in a patient with Wiskott-Aldrich syndrome." *Pediatr Blood Cancer* 59 (2):318-9. doi: 10.1002/pbc.23393.

[61] Kamani, N. R., S. Kumar, A. Hassebroek, M. Eapen, J. LeRademacher, J. Casper, M. Cowan, J. Sanchez de Toledo, A. Ferster, P. Szabolcs, J. R. Wingard, E. Horwitz, and A. H. Filipovich. 2011. "Malignancies after hematopoietic cell transplantation for primary immune deficiencies: a report from the Center for International Blood and Marrow Transplant Research."

Biol Blood Marrow Transplant 17 (12):1783-9. doi: 10.1016/j.bbmt.2011.05.008.

[62] Du, S., R. Scuderi, D. M. Malicki, J. Willert, J. Bastian, and N. Weidner. 2011. "Hodgkin's and non-Hodgkin's lymphomas occurring in two brothers with Wiskott-Aldrich syndrome and review of the literature." *Pediatr Dev Pathol* 14 (1):64-70. doi: 10.2350/10-01-0787-CR.1.

[63] Gangemi, S., A. Allegra, and C. Musolino. 2015. "Lymphoproliferative disease and cancer among patients with common variable immunodeficiency." *Leuk Res* 39 (4):389-96. doi: 10.1016/j.leukres.2015.02.002.

[64] Nelson, D. L., and C. Terhorst. 2000. "X-linked lymphoproliferative syndrome." *Clin Exp Immunol* 122 (3):291-5. doi: 10.1046/j.1365-2249.2000.01400.x.

[65] Rezaei, N., E. Mahmoudi, A. Aghamohammadi, R. Das, and K. E. Nichols. 2011. "X-linked lymphoproliferative syndrome: a genetic condition typified by the triad of infection, immunodeficiency and lymphoma." *Br J Haematol* 152 (1):13-30. doi: 10.1111/j.1365-2141.2010.08442.x.

[66] Sandlund, J. T., S. A. Shurtleff, M. Onciu, E. Horwitz, W. Leung, V. Howard, R. Rencher, and M. E. Conley. 2013. "Frequent mutations in SH2D1A (XLP) in males presenting with high-grade mature B-cell neoplasms." *Pediatr Blood Cancer* 60 (9):E85-7. doi: 10.1002/pbc.24525.

[67] Egeler, R. M., J. de Kraker, R. Slater, and D. T. Purtilo. 1992. "Documentation of Burkitt lymphoma with t(8;14) (q24;q32) in X-linked lymphoproliferative disease." *Cancer* 70 (3):683-7. doi: 10.1002/1097-0142(19920801)70:3<683::aid-cncr2820700324>3.0.co;2-c.

[68] Strahm, B., K. Rittweiler, U. Duffner, O. Brandau, M. Orlowska-Volk, M. A. Karajannis, Uz Stadt, M. Tiemann, A. Reiter, M. Brandis, A. Meindl, and C. M. Niemeyer. 2000. "Recurrent B-cell non-Hodgkin's lymphoma in two brothers with X-linked lymphoproliferative disease without evidence for Epstein-Barr virus

infection." *Br J Haematol* 108 (2):377-82. doi: 10.1046/j.1365-2141.2000.01884.x.

[69] Zhou, D., C. N. Paxton, T. W. Kelley, Z. Afify, S. T. South, and R. R. Miles. 2016. "Two Unrelated Burkitt Lymphomas Seven Years Apart in a Patient with X-Linked Lymphoproliferative Disease Type 1 (XLP1)." *Am J Clin Pathol* 146 (2):248-53. doi: 10.1093/ajcp/aqw036.

[70] Booth, C., K. C. Gilmour, P. Veys, A. R. Gennery, M. A. Slatter, H. Chapel, P. T. Heath, C. G. Steward, O. Smith, A. O'Meara, H. Kerrigan, N. Mahlaoui, M. Cavazzana-Calvo, A. Fischer, D. Moshous, S. Blanche, J. Pachlopnik Schmid, S. Latour, G. de Saint-Basile, M. Albert, G. Notheis, N. Rieber, B. Strahm, H. Ritterbusch, A. Lankester, N. G. Hartwig, I. Meyts, A. Plebani, A. Soresina, A. Finocchi, C. Pignata, E. Cirillo, S. Bonanomi, C. Peters, K. Kalwak, S. Pasic, P. Sedlacek, J. Jazbec, H. Kanegane, K. E. Nichols, I. C. Hanson, N. Kapoor, E. Haddad, M. Cowan, S. Choo, J. Smart, P. D. Arkwright, and H. B. Gaspar. 2011. "X-linked lymphoproliferative disease due to SAP/SH2D1A deficiency: a multicenter study on the manifestations, management and outcome of the disease." *Blood* 117 (1):53-62. doi: 10.1182/blood-2010-06-284935.

[71] Gilmour, K. C., and H. B. Gaspar. 2003. "Pathogenesis and diagnosis of X-linked lymphoproliferative disease." *Expert Rev Mol Diagn* 3 (5):549-61. doi: 10.1586/14737159.3.5.549.

[72] Brandau, O., V. Schuster, M. Weiss, H. Hellebrand, F. M. Fink, A. Kreczy, W. Friedrich, B. Strahm, C. Niemeyer, B. H. Belohradsky, and A. Meindl. 1999. "Epstein-Barr virus-negative boys with non-Hodgkin lymphoma are mutated in the SH2D1A gene, as are patients with X-linked lymphoproliferative disease (XLP)." *Hum Mol Genet* 8 (13):2407-13. doi: 10.1093/hmg/8.13.2407.

[73] Straus, S. E., E. S. Jaffe, J. M. Puck, J. K. Dale, K. B. Elkon, A. Rosen-Wolff, A. M. Peters, M. C. Sneller, C. W. Hallahan, J. Wang, R. E. Fischer, C. E. Jackson, A. Y. Lin, C. Baumler, E. Siegert, A. Marx, A. K. Vaishnaw, T. Grodzicky, T. A. Fleisher, and M. J. Lenardo. 2001. "The development of lymphomas in families with

autoimmune lymphoproliferative syndrome with germline Fas mutations and defective lymphocyte apoptosis." *Blood* 98 (1):194-200. doi: 10.1182/blood.v98.1.194.

[74] Afify, Z., E. Morales, A. Agarwal, K. Chen, and J. Bohnsack. "Diffuse large B-cell lymphoma (DLBCL) in a child with Di George syndrome." *British Journal of Hematology*, 2018:182, (Suppl), 142.

[75] Ramos, J. T., E. Lopez-Laso, J. Ruiz-Contreras, E. Giancaspro, and S. Madero. 1999. "B cell non-Hodgkin's lymphoma in a girl with the DiGeorge anomaly." *Arch Dis Child* 81 (5):444-5. doi: 10.1136/adc.81.5.444.

[76] Sato, T., O. Tatsuzawa, Y. Koike, Y. Wada, M. Nagata, S. Kobayashi, A. Ishizawa, J. Miyauchi, and K. Shimizu. "B-Cell Lymphoma Associated with Digeorge Syndrome." *Eur J Pediatr* 158, no. 7 (Jul 1999): 609. https://doi.org/10.1007/s004310051160.

[77] Hong, R., V. Shen, C. Rooney, D. P. Hughes, C. Smith, P. Comoli, and L. Zhang. 2001. "Correction of DiGeorge anomaly with EBV-induced lymphoma by transplantation of organ-cultured thymus and Epstein-Barr-specific cytotoxic T lymphocytes." *Clin Immunol* 98 (1):54-61. doi: 10.1006/clim.2000.4948.

[78] Loeb, D. M., H. M. Lederman, and J. A. Winkelstein. 2000. "Lymphoid malignancy as a presenting sign of ataxia-telangiectasia." *J Pediatr Hematol Oncol* 22 (5):464-7. doi: 10.1097/00043426-200009000-00017.

[79] Jastaniah, W. 2017. "Successful treatment of mature B-cell lymphoma with rituximab-based chemotherapy in a patient with Bloom syndrome." *Pediatr Blood Cancer* 64 (7). doi: 10.1002/pbc.26385.

[80] Dembowska-Baginska, B., D. Perek, A. Brozyna, A. Wakulinska, D. Olczak-Kowalczyk, M. Gladkowska-Dura, W. Grajkowska, and K. H. Chrzanowska. 2009. "Non-Hodgkin lymphoma (NHL) in children with Nijmegen Breakage syndrome (NBS)." *Pediatr Blood Cancer* 52 (2):186-90. doi: 10.1002/pbc.21789.

[81] Senapati, J., A. J. Devasia, S. David, M. T. Manipadam, S. Nair, G. R. Jayandharan, and B. George. 2014. "Diffuse large B cell

lymphoma in Wiskott-Aldrich syndrome: a case report and review of literature." *Indian J Hematol Blood Transfus* 30 (Suppl 1):309-13. doi: 10.1007/s12288-014-0377-1.

[82] Gilson, D., and R. E. Taylor. 1999. "Long-term survival following non-Hodgkin's lymphoma arising in Wiskott-Aldrich syndrome." *Clin Oncol (R Coll Radiol)* 11 (4):283-5. doi: 10.1053/clon.1999.9066.

[83] Palenzuela, G., F. Bernard, Q. Gardiner, and M. Mondain. 2003. "Malignant B cell non-Hodgkin's lymphoma of the larynx in children with Wiskott-Aldrich syndrome." *Int J Pediatr Otorhinolaryngol* 67 (9):989-93. doi: 10.1016/s0165-5876(03)00155-1.

[84] Nakanishi, M., H. Kikuta, K. Tomizawa, K. Kojima, A. Ishizaka, M. Okano, Y. Sakiyama, and S. Matsumoto. 1993. "Distinct clonotypic Epstein-Barr virus-induced fatal lymphoproliferative disorder in a patient with Wiskott-Aldrich syndrome." *Cancer* 72 (4):1376-81. doi: 10.1002/1097-0142(19930815)72:4<1376::aid-cncr2820720437>3.0.co;2-q.

[85] Cunningham, D., E. A. Hawkes, A. Jack, W. Qian, P. Smith, P. Mouncey, C. Pocock, K. M. Ardeshna, J. A. Radford, A. McMillan, J. Davies, D. Turner, A. Kruger, P. Johnson, J. Gambell, and D. Linch. 2013. "Rituximab plus cyclophosphamide, doxorubicin, vincristine, and prednisolone in patients with newly diagnosed diffuse large B-cell non-Hodgkin lymphoma: a phase 3 comparison of dose intensification with 14-day versus 21-day cycles." *Lancet* 381 (9880):1817-26. doi: 10.1016/S0140-6736(13)60313-X.

[86] Coiffier, B., C. Thieblemont, E. Van Den Neste, G. Lepeu, I. Plantier, S. Castaigne, S. Lefort, G. Marit, M. Macro, C. Sebban, K. Belhadj, D. Bordessoule, C. Ferme, and H. Tilly. 2010. "Long-term outcome of patients in the LNH-98.5 trial, the first randomized study comparing rituximab-CHOP to standard CHOP chemotherapy in DLBCL patients: a study by the Groupe d'Etudes des Lymphomes de l'Adulte." *Blood* 116 (12):2040-5. doi: 10.1182/blood-2010-03-276246.

[87] Coiffier, B., E. Lepage, J. Briere, R. Herbrecht, H. Tilly, R. Bouabdallah, P. Morel, E. Van Den Neste, G. Salles, P. Gaulard, F. Reyes, P. Lederlin, and C. Gisselbrecht. 2002. "CHOP chemotherapy plus rituximab compared with CHOP alone in elderly patients with diffuse large-B-cell lymphoma." *N Engl J Med* 346 (4):235-42. doi: 10.1056/NEJMoa011795.

[88] Luo, C., G. Wu, X. Huang, Y. Ma, Y. Zhang, Q. Song, M. Xie, Y. Sun, Y. Huang, Z. Huang, Y. Hou, S. Xu, J. Chen, and X. Li. 2021. "Efficacy and safety of new anti-CD20 monoclonal antibodies versus rituximab for induction therapy of CD20(+) B-cell non-Hodgkin lymphomas: a systematic review and meta-analysis." *Sci Rep* 11 (1):3255. doi: 10.1038/s41598-021-82841-w.

[89] Hutchings, M., C. Carlo-Stella, M. Bachy, F. Offner, M. Morschhauser, F. Crump, M. Iacoboni, A. Sureda Balari, J. Martinez-Lopez, L. Lundberg, M., Dixon, D. Perez Callejo, J. Relf, D. Carlile, E. Piccione, K. Humphrey, and M. Dickinson. "Glofitamab Step-up Dosing Induces High Response Rates in Patients with Hard-to-Treat Refractory or Relapsed Non-Hodgkin Lymphoma". *American Society of Hematology* 2020. Abstract 403.

[90] Schuster, S. J., J. Svoboda, E. A. Chong, S. D. Nasta, A. R. Mato, O. Anak, J. L. Brogdon, I. Pruteanu-Malinici, V. Bhoj, D. Landsburg, M. Wasik, B. L. Levine, S. F. Lacey, J. J. Melenhorst, D. L. Porter, and C. H. June. 2017. "Chimeric Antigen Receptor T Cells in Refractory B-Cell Lymphomas." *N Engl J Med* 377 (26):2545-2554. doi: 10.1056/NEJMoa1708566.

[91] Strati, P., A. Varma, S. Adkins, L. J. Nastoupil, J. Westin, F. B. Hagemeister, N. H. Fowler, H. J. Lee, L. E. Fayad, F. Samaniego, S. Ahmed, Y. Chen, S. Horowitz, S. Arafat, S. Johncy, P. Kebriaei, V. E. Mulanovich, E. Ariza Heredia, and S. S. Neelapu. 2020. "Hematopoietic recovery and immune reconstitution after axicabtagene ciloleucel in patients with large B-cell lymphoma." *Haematologica.* doi: 10.3324/haematol.2020.254045.

[92] Locke, F. L., A. Ghobadi, C. A. Jacobson, D. B. Miklos, L. J. Lekakis, O. O. Oluwole, Y. Lin, I. Braunschweig, B. T. Hill, J. M.

Timmerman, A. Deol, P. M. Reagan, P. Stiff, I. W. Flinn, U. Farooq, A. Goy, P. A. McSweeney, J. Munoz, T. Siddiqi, J. C. Chavez, A. F. Herrera, N. L. Bartlett, J. S. Wiezorek, L. Navale, A. Xue, Y. Jiang, A. Bot, J. M. Rossi, J. J. Kim, W. Y. Go, and S. S. Neelapu. 2019. “Long-term safety and activity of axicabtagene ciloleucel in refractory large B-cell lymphoma (ZUMA-1): a single-arm, multicentre, phase 1-2 trial.” *Lancet Oncol* 20 (1):31-42. doi: 10.1016/S1470-2045(18)30864-7

[93] Maude, S. L., N. Frey, P. A. Shaw, R. Aplenc, D. M. Barrett, N. J. Bunin, A. Chew, V. E. Gonzalez, Z. Zheng, S. F. Lacey, Y. D. Mahnke, J. J. Melenhorst, S. R. Rheingold, A. Shen, D. T. Teachey, B. L. Levine, C. H. June, D. L. Porter, and S. A. Grupp. 2014. “Chimeric antigen receptor T cells for sustained remissions in leukemia.” *N Engl J Med* 371 (16):1507-17. doi: 10.1056/NEJMoa1407222.

[94] Zeng, C., J. Cheng, T. Li, J. Huang, C. Li, L. Jiang, J. Wang, L. Chen, X. Mao, L. Zhu, Y. Lou, J. Zhou, and X. Zhou. 2020. “Efficacy and toxicity for CD22/CD19 chimeric antigen receptor T-cell therapy in patients with relapsed/refractory aggressive B-cell lymphoma involving the gastrointestinal tract.” *Cytotherapy* 22 (3):166-171. doi: 10.1016/j.jcyt.2020.01.008.

[95] Avigdor, A., R. Shouval, E. Jacoby, T. Davidson, A. Shimoni, M. Besser, and A. Nagler. 2018. “CAR T cells induce a complete response in refractory Burkitt Lymphoma.” *Bone Marrow Transplant* 53 (12):1583-1585. doi: 10.1038/s41409-018-0235-0.

[96] Du, J., and Y. Zhang. 2020. “Correction to: Sequential anti-CD19, 22, and 20 autologous chimeric antigen receptor T-cell (CAR-T) treatments of a child with relapsed refractory Burkitt lymphoma: a case report and literature review.” *J Cancer Res Clin Oncol* 146 (8):2177. doi: 10.1007/s00432-020-03269-9.

[97] Bollard, C. M., S. Gottschalk, V. Torrano, O. Diouf, S. Ku, Y. Hazrat, G. Carrum, C. Ramos, L. Fayad, E. J. Shpall, B. Pro, H. Liu, M. F. Wu, D. Lee, A. M. Sheehan, Y. Zu, A. P. Gee, M. K. Brenner, H. E. Heslop, and C. M. Rooney. 2014. “Sustained complete

responses in patients with lymphoma receiving autologous cytotoxic T lymphocytes targeting Epstein-Barr virus latent membrane proteins." *J Clin Oncol* 32 (8):798-808. doi: 10.1200/JCO.2013.51.5304.

[98] Dalton, T., E. Doubrovina, D. Pankov, R. Reynolds, H. Scholze, A. Selvakumar, T. Vizconde, B. Savalia, V. Dyomin, C. Weigel, C. C. Oakes, A. Alonso, O. Elemento, H. Pan, J. M. Phillip, R. J. O'Reilly, B. E. Gewurz, E. Cesarman, and L. Giulino-Roth. 2020. "Epigenetic reprogramming sensitizes immunologically silent EBV+ lymphomas to virus-directed immunotherapy." *Blood* 135 (21):1870-1881. doi: 10.1182/blood.2019004126.

[99] Albert, M. H., A. R. Gennery, J. Greil, C. M. Cale, K. Kalwak, I. Kondratenko, W. Mlynarski, G. Notheis, M. Fuhrer, I. Schmid, and B. H. Belohradsky. 2010. "Successful SCT for Nijmegen breakage syndrome." *Bone Marrow Transplant* 45 (4):622-6. doi: 10.1038/bmt.2009.207.

[100] Slack, J., M. H. Albert, D. Balashov, B. H. Belohradsky, A. Bertaina, J. Bleesing, C. Booth, J. Buechner, R. H. Buckley, M. Ouachee-Chardin, E. Deripapa, K. Drabko, M. Eapen, T. Feuchtinger, A. Finocchi, H. B. Gaspar, S. Ghosh, A. Gillio, L. I. Gonzalez-Granado, E. Grunebaum, T. Gungor, C. Heilmann, M. Helminen, K. Higuchi, K. Imai, K. Kalwak, N. Kanazawa, G. Karasu, Z. Y. Kucuk, A. Laberko, A. Lange, N. Mahlaoui, R. Meisel, D. Moshous, H. Muramatsu, S. Parikh, S. Pasic, I. Schmid, C. Schuetz, A. Schulz, K. R. Schultz, P. J. Shaw, M. A. Slatter, K. W. Sykora, S. Tamura, M. Taskinen, A. Wawer, B. Wolska-Kusnierz, M. J. Cowan, A. Fischer, A. R. Gennery, Blood Inborn Errors Working Party of the European Society for, Transplantation Marrow, Immunodeficiencies the European Society for, Europe Stem Cell Transplant for Immunodeficiencies in, Blood Center for International, Research Marrow Transplant, and Consortium Primary Immunodeficiency Treatment. 2018. "Outcome of hematopoietic cell transplantation for DNA double-strand break

repair disorders." *J Allergy Clin Immunol* 141 (1):322-328 e10. doi: 10.1016/j.jaci.2017.02.036.

[101] Bhatt, J. M., Bush, A., van Gerven, M., Nissenkorn, A., Renke, M., Yarlett, L., Taylor, M., Tonia, T., Warris, A., Zielen, S., Zinna, S., and Merkus, P. J. 2015. "*Ataxia telangiectasia*: why should the ERS care?" *Eur Respir J* 46 (6):1557-60. doi: 10.1183/13993003.01456-2015.

[102] German, J. 1997. "Bloom's syndrome. XX. The first 100 cancers." *Cancer Genet Cytogenet* 93 (1):100-6. doi: 10.1016/s0165-4608(96)00336-6.

[103] Martin-Mateos, M. A., and M. Piquer Gibert. 2016. "Primary immunodeficiencies and B-cell lymphomas." *Bol Med Hosp Infant Mex* 73 (1):18-25. doi: 10.1016/j.bmhimx.2015.11.009.

[104] Danby, C. S., L. Allen, M. D. Moharir, S. Weitzman, and T. Dumont. 2013. "Non-hodgkin B-cell lymphoma of the ovary in a child with Ataxia-telangiectasia." *J Pediatr Adolesc Gynecol* 26 (2):e43-5. doi: 10.1016/j.jpag.2012.09.003.

[105] Fedorova, A., S. Sharapova, T. Mikhalevskaya, S. Aleshkevich, I. Proleskovskaya, M. Belevtsev, and O. Aleinikova. 2015. "Non-Hodgkin Lymphoma in Children with Primary Immunodeficiencies: Clinical Manifestations, Diagnosis, and Management, Belarusian Experience." *Lymphoma* 2015:1-10. doi: 10.1155/2015/123548.

Biographical Sketch

Zeinab A. Afify

Affiliation: Associate Professor, Pediatric Hematology/ Oncology, University Of Utah

Education:

1997 - 1998	Clinical Fellow	Children's Hospital of Westmead -Pediatric Oncology and Bone Marrow Transplantation, Sydney, NSW, Australia
1996	Senior Registrar	Alder Hey Children's Hospital, Liverpool, United Kingdom
1994 - 1995	Resident	Riley Hospital for Children-Pediatrics, Indianapolis, IN
1993 - 1994	Clinical Fellow	Riley Hospital for Children -Pediatric Hematology/Oncology, Indianapolis, IN
1992 - 1993	Clinical Fellow	University of Iowa Hospitals and Clinics - Pediatric Hematology/Oncology, Iowa City, IA
1988 - 1989	Research Fellow	Emory University School of Medicine - Pediatric Hematology/Oncology, Atlanta, GA
1983 - 1986	Resident	University of Alexandria Children's Hospital -Pediatrics, Alexandria, Egypt
1981 - 1982	Intern	University of Alexandria Hospitals, Alexandria, Egypt
1974 - 1980	M.B.B.Ch.	University of Alexandria -Medicine, Alexandria, Egypt

Professional Appointments and Experience:

2008 - Present	Associate Professor, Pediatric Hematology/Oncology, University of Utah, Salt Lake City, UT
2002 - 2008	Assistant Professor, Pediatric Hematology/Oncology, University of Utah, Salt Lake City, UT
2002	Locum Consultant Pediatric Oncologist, Llandough Hospital, Cardiff, United Kingdom

2002	Elective Subspecialty Clinical Fellowship in Stem Cell Transplantation (SCT), Bristol Royal Hospital for Sick Children, Bristol, United Kingdom
2001	Consultant Pediatric Hematologist Oncologist, Locum, Royal Children's Hospital, Pediatric Hematology/Oncology and SCT Unit, Brisbane, Australia
1998 - 2001	Pediatric Hematologist/Oncologist, Tawam Hospital, Department of Pediatrics, Al Ain, United Arab Emirates.
1995 - 1996	Lecturer of Pediatrics, University of Alexandria Children Hospital, Department of Pediatrics, Alexandria, Egypt
1990 - 1992	Lecturer of Pediatrics, University of Alexandria Children Hospital, Department of Pediatrics, Alexandria, Egypt
1986 - 1990	Assistant Lecturer of Pediatrics, University of Alexandria Children Hospital, Department of Pediatrics, Alexandria, Egypt

Research Experience:

Clinical Studies

2021 - Present	Institutional Principal Investigator: LCH-IV International study of North American Consortium of Histiocytic Disorders (NACHO). The study consists of 7 clinical strata of pediatric patients with Langerhans cell histiocytosis. Under local regulatory review, expected to open fall, 2021
2021 - Present	Institutional Principal Investigator: NACHO BIO: A study of the biology of pediatric histiocytic disorders. Under local regulatory review.

2020 - Present	Investigator-Initiated Study: Retrospective multi-center study evaluating clinical and pathological features, risk factors and outcome of children with post-solid organ transplant monomorphic lymphoproliferative disease (M-PTLD) including Burkitt lymphoma (BL).
2020 - Present	Coinvestigator, Children's Oncology Group (COG) Study. Blinatumomab and R-ICE chemotherapy in relapsed refractory mature B cell non-Hodgkin lymphoma (B-NHL)-under development, expected to open 2021/2022.
2019 - 2020	Institutional Principal Investigator, MHE112562/01, Expanded access to mepolizumab for patients with hypereosinophilic syndrome, Industry Sponsored
2018	Institutional Principal Investigator, Single Patient Use IND - Ruxolitinib, Industry Sponsored
2016 - 2017	Co-investigator, University of Utah study: Variable expressivity and incomplete penetrance in a large family with non-classical Diamond-Blackfan anemia associated with ribosomal protein L11 splicing variant
2016 - 2017	Co-investigator: Outcomes of adults and children with primary mediastinal B-Cell lymphoma treated with dose-adjusted EPOCH-R
2014 - 2016	Co-investigator, University of Utah study: Two unrelated Burkitt lymphomas seven years apart in a patient with X- linked lymphoproliferative disease Type 1 (XLP1).
2010 - 2011	Co-investigator, University of Utah study: Clinicopathologic comparison of familial versus sporadic Atypical Teratoid/ Rhabdoid Tumors (AT/RT) of the central nervous system: the Utah experience.
2007 - 2009	Co-Investigator Children's Oncology GroupANHL06P1- A Phase I/II Pilot, Study of ICE and SGN-30 in children with CD30 positive recurrent anaplastic large cell lymphomas (ALCL)

2004 - 2016	Co-Investigator, Children's Oncology Group Study ANHL04B1 - Rare and Cutaneous Non-Hodgkin Lymphoma Registry

Independent Research

2020 - 2021	Role: Principal Investigator Project Title: Diffuse large B-cell lymphoma (DLBCL) in DiGeorge syndrome. Scope: Two-institution study in collaboration with All Children's Hospital, Saint Petersburg, FL. Description: A study of clinical features and therapy outcome in the rare association of lymphoma and Di George syndrome. Manuscript in progress.
2020 - Present	Role: Principal Investigator Project Title: High index of suspicion for lymphoma can guide a conservative surgical approach to Abdominal mass presentation. Scope: Institutional study Description. A study of the impact of the extent of initial biopsy on outcome of children presenting with abdominal mass with lymphomatous features. Study in progress
2019 - 2020	Role: Principal Investigator Project Title: Two clonally distinct B-cell lymphomas reveal the diagnosis of XLP1 in a male child and his asymptomatic male relatives. Scope: Institutional study Description: A study of role of clonality testing to diagnose 2 separate lymphomas rather than recurrent lymphoma in patients suspected to have X-linked lymphoproliferative disease. Published
2019 - 2020	Role: Co-Investigator Scope: Institutional study Project Title: Postnatal monitoring of hyporegenerative anemia following intrauterine transfusions for Rh-D allo-immunizations Description: The findings are expected to increase knowledge of this important clinical entity and improve preventive measures, management and outcome. Accepted for publication 2021

2018 - 2020	Role: Principal Investigator Project Title: Complete blood count analysis can eliminate the need for biopsy in some children with new onset B-acute lymphoblastic leukemia presenting with an extramedullary mass. Scope: Institutional study Description: The study is expected to impact clinical practice in these patients by early communication between referring pediatricians, surgeons and pediatric oncologists to minimize invasive investigations. Manuscript in progress
2018 - 2020	Role: Co-iInvestigator Project Title: Clinical spectrum and management of immune cytopenias in children with partial DiGeorge syndrome Scope: Two-institution study in collaboration with All Children's Hospital, Saint Petersburg, FL. Description: This study expands knowledge of therapeutic options for autoimmune cytopenias in patients with DiGeorge syndrome based on clinical severity and response to treatment. Manuscript in progress
2014 - 2016	Role: Principal Investigator Scope: University of Utah study Project Title: Pediatric B- cell lymphoma with lymphoblastic morphology, TdT expression, MYC rearrangement, and features overlapping with Burkitt Lymphoma Description: This study provided evidence of clinical efficacy of an intensive regimen in a unique and seldom studied type of NHL combining features of 2 lymphoma subtypes. Published

Publications from the Last 3 Years:

1. El-Atoum, B., Ebert, M., Bucher, B., Afify, Z. (2021). Is 18F-FDG PET/CT effective in identifying true residual disease after treatment of pediatric PTLD? [Letter to the editor]. Accepted for publication 2021 in *The Journal of Nuclear Medicine*.

2. Thomsen, C. W., Afify, Z. Late Hyporegenerative Anemia Following Successful Management of Rh-D Alloimmunization: Still An Underappreciated Entity. Accepted for publication in *Clinical Pediatrics* 2021.
3. Iglesias Cardenas, F., Agarwal, A. M., Vagher, J., Maese, L., Fluchel, M., Afify, Z. (2021). Two Clonally Distinct B-Cell Lymphomas Reveal the Diagnosis of XLP1 in a Male Child and His Asymptomatic Male Relatives: Case Report and Review of the Literature. (Epub ahead of print) *J Pediatr Hematol Oncol*.
4. Carter Febres, M., Abbott, J., Cipriano, S. D., Knackstedt, E. D., George, T. I., Afify, Z. (2021). Drug reaction with eosinophilia and systemic symptoms (DRESS)-associated hemophagocytic lymphohistiocytosis (HLH), an important and underrecognized HLH mimic: A case report. [Letter to the editor]. *Pediatr Blood Cancer*, *68*(2), e28657.
5. Febres, M. C., Viskochil, D., Rampton, J., Afify, Z. (2020). Further Lessons Learned From a Child With NF1 and Classical Hodgkin Lymphoma. [Letter to the editor]. *J Pediatr Hematol Oncol*.
6. Carter-Febres, M., Smock, K. J., Ware, A. L., Afify, Z. A. (2020). Improvement of Bleeding Manifestations of Acquired Von Willebrand Syndrome after Balloon Aortic Valvoplasty in a child with Aortic Stenosis. https://doi.org/10.1016/j.ppedcard.2020.101334. *Prog Ped Cardiol*.
7. Giulino-Roth, L., O'Donohue, T., Chen, Z., Bartlett, N. L., LaCasce, A., Martin-Doyle, W., Barth, M. J., Davies, K., Blum, K. A., Christian, B., Casulo, C., Smith, S. M., Godfrey, J., Termuhlen, A., Oberley, M. J., Alexander, S., Weitzman, S., Appel, B., Mizukawa, B., Svoboda, J., Afify, Z., Pauly, M., Dave, H., Gardner, R., Stephens, D. M., Zeitler, W. A., Forlenza, C., Levine, J., Williams, M. E., Sima, J. L., Bollard, C. M., Leonard, J. P. (2017). Outcomes of adults and children with primary mediastinal B-cell lymphoma treated with dose-adjusted EPOCH-R. *Br J Haematol*, *179*(5), 739-747.

8. Carlston, C. M., Afify, Z. A., Palumbos, J. C., Bagley, H., Barbagelata, C., Wooderchak-Donahue, W. L., Mao, R., Carey, J. C. (2017). Variable expressivity and incomplete penetrance in a large family with non-classical Diamond-Blackfan anemia associated with ribosomal protein L11 splicing variant. *Am J Med Genet A*, *173*(10), 2622-2627.
9. Maese, L., Li, K. D., Xu, X., Afify, Z., Paxton, C. N., Putnam, A. (2017). . Acute Leukemia and Concurrent Mediastinal Germ Cell Tumor: Case Report and Literature Review. [Review]. *Fetal Pediatr Pathol*, *36*(2), 168-176.
10. Gallagher-Lacey, C., Afify, Z., Yaish, H. M., Yoder, B. A., Christensen, R. D. (2017). An Instructive Case of Transient Myeloproliferative Disorder. *Clin Pediatr (Phila)*, *56*(3), 288-289.
11. Zhou, D., Paxton, C. N., Kelley, T. W., Afify, Z., South, S .T., Miles, R. R. (2016). Two Unrelated Burkitt Lymphomas Seven Years Apart in a Patient with X-Linked Lymphoproliferative Disease Type 1 (XLP1). *Am J Clin Pathol*, *146*(2), 248-53.
12. Meznarich, J., Miles, R., Paxton, C. N., Afify, Z. (2016). Pediatric B-Cell Lymphoma with Lymphoblastic Morphology, TdT Expression, MYC Rearrangement, and Features Overlapping With Burkitt Lymphoma. *Pediatr Blood Cancer*, *63*(5), 938-40.

In: Burkitt Lymphoma
Editor: Douglas V. Berthelot
ISBN: 978-1-68507-071-7

Chapter 3

POST SOLID ORGAN TRANSPLANT BURKITT LYMPHOMA

***Zeinab Afify*[1,*] *and Angela Punnett*[2]**
[1]Division of Hematology/Oncology, Department of Pediatrics, University of Utah, Salt Lake City, Utah, US
[2]Department of Pediatrics, University of Toronto and SickKids Hospital, Toronto, Ontario, Canada

ABSTRACT

The incidence of Burkitt lymphoma (BL) is markedly elevated in solid organ transplant recipients compared to the general population. It is frequently a late event occurring more than 1-2 years after transplantation. This in contrast to other forms of post-transplant lymphoproliferative disorders (PTLD), the majority of which occur in the first year after transplantation. Post solid organ transplant Burkitt lymphoma (PSOT-BL) is most often Epstein Barr virus (EBV) positive, in contrast to sporadic BL (sBL) in immunocompetent patients (IC-BL). It differs from other forms of monomorphic post-transplant

* Corresponding Author's E-mail: Zeinab.afify@imail.org.

lymphoproliferative disorders (M-PTLD) with a distinct pathologic and molecular profile.

There is no defined standard treatment regimen for PSOT-BL and both adult and pediatric studies have used approaches ranging from low dose chemotherapy regimens with or without the addition of rituximab to more intensive immunochemotherapeutic regimens similar to those used for IC-BL. The latter approach appears to be more effective, though treatment related morbidity and mortality remain major limitations, particularly in older patients. Of particular concern are the risk of infection related death, risk of rejection and higher risk of end organ toxicities specific to the allograft. Guidelines for treatment modification and data on the impact on survival, graft function or long-term toxicity are lacking.

In this chapter we will review the incidence, clinicopathological and epidemiologic features, treatment and outcome data available in pediatric and adult patients with PSOT-BL. Finally we will focus on specific treatment considerations and the unique challenges in designing regimens based on the organ transplanted and patient comorbidities.

Keywords: Burkitt lymphoma, solid organ transplantation, immune-suppression, Epstein-Barr virus, non-Hodgkin lymphoma

1. Introduction

Post solid organ transplant Burkitt lymphoma (PSOT-BL) is a late form of monomorphic post-transplant lymphoproliferative disorder (M-PTLD) with an aggressive clinical presentation and distinct pathologic profile. Compared to the general population, the incidence of Burkitt lymphoma is increased 23-fold in solid organ transplant recipients [1] though it is relatively uncommon compared to the development of other types of M-PTLD, including diffuse large B-cell lymphoma (DLBCL) [1, 2]. Published data about treatment, treatment related morbidity and mortality are limited by the small number of patients with PSOT-BL [1-7]. Patients are most often included in studies or series of M- PTLD more broadly, with limited BL specific treatment and outcome data [3-6]. Therefore, the optimal therapy in PSOT-BL remains unclear.

2. Epidemiology

With the steady growth of the use of solid organ transplantation over the past 30 years [1, 2] combined with improved transplant outcomes, cancer is becoming an increasing problem for transplant recipients [1]. Post-transplant lymphoproliferative disease contributes 3% of all pediatric non-Hodgkin lymphoma (NHL) diagnoses of the nearly 1040 new cases of NHL diagnosed annually in US [8]. The incidence of pediatric NHL/PTLD was reported by Yanik et al. to be 212 times higher than the general population [2]. The majority (65%) of NHL/PTLD cases are DLBCLs; and less than 10% of cases are BL [2, 8]

A large NIH study provides the most comprehensive incidence and demographic data available for PSOT-BL. The US Transplant Cancer Match (TCM Study) utilized linked data from the Scientific Registry of Transplant Recipients (SRTR) and population-based cancer registries in 15 states and/or metropolitan areas in USA. The study investigated the incidence of BL from 1987–2009 in 203,557 solid organ recipients and compared it to the general population using standardized incidence ratios (SIRs), and assessed associations with demographic, clinical characteristics, and type of immunosuppression used. The incidence of PSOT-BL was 10.8 per 100,000 person-years, representing a 23-fold (95% CI 19–28) greater risk than in the general population [1]. A similar SIR of 24.5 was reported by Clarke et al. [9].

Gender and race/ethnicity impact the incidence of PSOT-BL. The incidence of PSOT-BL in females was half that observed among males $P<0.001$; incidence rate ratio (IRR) 0.45, 95% CI 0.28–0.71) [1]. This is similar to the gender difference noted in endemic BL (eBL) [10], but less marked than the difference noted in IC-BL (4.5:1 male to female) [10, 11]. In a study by the French Society of Pediatric Oncology (SFOP), of 17 patients with PSOT-BL 12 were male [12]. In the TCM Study, the incidence of PSOT-BL was a third in blacks compared to whites (IRR 0.33, 95% CI 0.12–0.74). The rate among Hispanics and Asians/Pacific Islanders was similar to that in whites [1].

2.1. Demographic Risk Factors

The incidence of PSOT-BL is reported to be inversely related to age at transplantation. The TCM Study reported an IRR of 3.49 for recipients transplanted <18 vs. ≥35 years (95% CI 2.08–5.68) [1]. Among recipients aged less than 20 years at the time of transplantation, the risk was strikingly elevated for BL (SIR 123, 95% CI: 79.0–183) [2]. The increased susceptibility of the pediatric population to PTLD, including PSOT-BL can be partly explained by the higher rate of pre-transplant EBV seronegativity compared to adults [13]. The TCM Study reported a lower incidence of PSOT-BL among those with a baseline Epstein-Barr virus (EBV)-seropositive versus EBV-seronegative status (IRR 0.34, 95% CI 0.13–0.93) [1].

2.2. Transplant Risk Factors

Compared to other forms of PTLD, the development of PSOT-BL appears to be a late occurring event, after the first one to two years from transplantation and beyond [1, 12]. In contrast, 75% of other forms develop in the first year after solid organ transplantation (SOT).[3] In the TCM study the incidence was low in the first two years after transplantation, but rose steeply in the third year and remained elevated for 3–8 years after transplantation; (IRR 1.73, 95% CI 1.09-2.70) [1]. Similarly, in the study of 17 pediatric patients by Cohen-Cogo et al., median time to the onset of PSOT-BL was 3.4 years post-transplantation (range: 1.3-13.0) [12].

The influence of organ transplanted on the incidence of PSOT-BL were reported by Clarke et al. Standardized incidence ratios were highest in liver followed by heart and/or lung, and kidney recipients, with SIRs of 47.1, 33.0, 14.7 respectively [9]. Similarly, the TCM Study reported the risk of PSOT-BL to be higher in recipients transplanted with liver, IRR 2.91, (95% CI 1.68–5.09), or heart, IRR 2.39 (95% CI 1.30–4.31) compared to kidney [1].

The TCM Study did not find a significantly increased risk of PSOT-BL with the use of calcineurin inhibitors and noted a marginal decrease in risk among those recipients treated with azathioprine (IRR 0.69, 95% CI 0.43–1.07) and significantly decreased risk among those treated with mycophenolate mofetil (0.64, 95% CI 0.41–0.96) or corticosteroids (0.47, 95% CI 0.29–0.80) [1].

3. Biopathology

3.1. Pathologic and Genetic Features

Endemic and sporadic BL are recognized by the World Health organization as distinct entities [14], but are histologically indistinguishable. Both are associated with the translocation of the c-MYC proto-oncogene on chromosome 8 (8q24) to the heavy or light chain immunoglobulin loci on chromosome 14q32 (80% of cases), and less frequently 2p12, or 22q11 [10, 15-17], albeit with varying breakpoints [18]. In PSOT-BL c-MYC translocation is considered an early event that plays a primary role in pathogenesis of the process of malignant transformation that involves a B-cell-specific DNA modification mechanism [19]. In 2 studies of adult patients with the PSOT-BL, all tumors were positive for MYC translocations (a total of five in one study and seven in the other) [19, 20]. Piccaluga et al. found that three BL subtypes, sporadic, endemic and human immunodeficiency virus-positive, share a common gene expression signature, distinct from other B-cell malignancies, and suggested that not EBV, but the MYC-dependent signature had a major effect on the clustering [21]. More recently studies of 59 molecularly defined BL identified a novel aberration manifested by a specific 11q-gain/loss pattern in two cases (3%) lacking the MYC translocation [22]. Subsequently, in a study by Ferreiro et al., this peculiar 11q-gain/loss aberration was reported to be particularly frequent in BL in immunodeficient hosts, as it was identified in three of seven patients with

PSOT-BL receiving immunosuppressive maintenance therapy. Interestingly all three MYC translocation negative cases were also EBV negative. In order to identify the genes affected by the 11q imbalances, they compared gene expression profiles of the four cases with 11q-gain/loss, with the four MYC translocation positive cases. Altogether, 33 genes with a differential expression were identified. There was lower expression of MYC mRNA in PSOT-BL cases with the 11q-gain/loss pattern compared to the cases that were MYC-translocation positive. Hierarchical clustering of the studied cases using the set of 11q23/q24 dysregulated genes showed that MYC translocation-negative PSOT-BL cases cluster together and separately from MYC-translocation-positive PSOT-BL cases. To unravel the biological consequences of the 11q-gain/loss aberration in BL, they used Ingenuity Pathway Analysis, which showed that the genes are implicated in important biological processes, including cancer, and the majority of them (22/33) are involved in the TP53 and MYC networks, frequently by direct protein-protein interactions. These findings and the observation that cases with 11q imbalances cluster with MYC-translocation-positive BL suggest that the 11q-gain/loss aberration is a molecular variant of t(8q24/MYC) affecting the same or overlapping pathological pathways. They concluded that this aberration is more frequent in BL occurring in the setting of PSOT-BL (40-60%) than in IC-BL (3%), and proposed that immunosuppression may favor its formation. Because of the small number with PSOT-BL in this study they suggested that further studies of PSOT-BL are needed to explore this potential association further [23].

3.2. The Role of EBV in PTLD and PSOT-BL

Epstein-Barr virus is a risk factor for the development of PTLD and PSOT-BL. Circulating B lymphocytes latently infected with EBV are normally controlled by EBV-specific cytotoxic T cells (CTL) directed against latent viral proteins. The T cell suppression required to prevent allograft rejection among solid organ transplant recipients may lead to uncontrolled proliferation of EBV-positive B cells [24, 25]. Children have an elevated risk because, in contrast to adults, they are often EBV-naïve before transplantation and acquire EBV infection after transplantation [13]. In PSOT-BL, Burkitt cells express latent viral proteins that are targets for CTLs, but are able to survive and proliferate because of the lack of CTL activity [26]. Epstein-Barr virus infected B cells can persist in the germinal center where they are prone to somatic hypermutation, alteration of Bcl2 and MYC expression and activation of NF-kB/Bcl2/mTOR pathways, driving lymphocyte proliferation [27]. The accumulation of additional genetic defects transforms EBV-positive B cells to atypical lymphoproliferation. Classic transforming events that contribute to lymphomagenesis in immunocompetent individuals, such as chromosomal translocations [10], seem to add more to the pathogenesis of late PTLD development, which more often results in distinct entities as in PSOT-BL [28]. With more advanced tools to detect genetic alterations such as whole-genome sequencing, our understanding of PTLD development by sequential genetic 'hits' will likely greatly improve [13].

Epstein-Barr virus is detected more frequently in pediatric PSOT-BL. In the TCM study, EBV was positive in 69% of tumors in 32 cases with EBV results available including 90% in those <18 years of age and 59% in those > 18 years [1]. In earlier case reports and case series of PSOT-BL, EBV was detected in the majority but not all PSOT-BL [7, 19, 20, 26, 29-34]. In comparison, EBV is detected in nearly 95% of e-BL tumors and only 20-30% of sporadic BL in immunocompetent patients [8, 10]. The prognostic significance of EBV negativity in PSOT-BL is currently unknown.

3.3. Epstein-Barr Virus DNAemia Load

Based on the understanding that naive B lymphocyte infection results in the differentiation of EBV-infected B cells and the potential for developing lymphoproliferative disease in patients with cellular immune defects [35], it is hypothesized that increasing EBV DNA load in the blood may be diagnostic of or precede PTLD disease [36]. However, the relationship of EBV DNAemia load, its monitoring and the development of PTLD in SOT recipients is complex [37]. Typically, primary EBV replication in a seronegative SOT recipient is associated with a higher risk of PTLD [13, 38]. On the other hand, EBV DNAemia detection is common after SOT and does not seem to be per se consistently related to the development of PTLD. Chronic or persistent high EBV load carriers (defined as chronic high-load state of >16 000 genome copies/mL whole blood on ≥50% of samples over at least 6 months) [39] are not clearly related to higher risk of the development of EBV-positive PTLD [36]. Given the lack of consensus on a static threshold EBV load for preemptive intervention [36], some authors have suggested that the rise in EBV load may be more informative about the risk of developing PTLD [37, 40]. For patients with risk factors for development of PTLD including EBV seronegative recipients, those in whom T-cell depleting antibodies were used, or those with rising viral loads, judicious escalation of interventions based on EBV load monitoring such as reducing immunosuppression and radiological surveillance for PTLD, should be considered [36].

4. Clinical Features and Involved Sites

Nodal presentation is most common in PSOT-BL, reported in 75% of cases and widely distributed anatomically. Extranodal sites were most commonly abdominal including small or large intestine and liver. Other extranodal sites were less commonly reported and include bone marrow (4%), and miscellaneous sites such as the nasopharynx, mediastinum, spinal cord/meninges, and soft tissue (5%) [1]. Bone marrow involvement and CNS involvement were much higher in a pediatric study of 17 patients with PSOT-BL at 40% and 11% respectively [12]. This latter experience is more in keeping with the pediatric experience for IC-BL [41].

5. Treatment

5.1. Are Treatment Strategies for M-PTLD Effective in BL?

Patients with M-PTLD may respond to reduction of immunosuppression (RIS) and/or specific anti-B cell immunotherapy (rituximab). Response-based treatment approach has been adopted by several groups with good outcomes. The use of chemotherapy is often reserved for patients with inadequate response to RIS and to rituximab [3, 42, 43]. The most commonly used chemotherapy regimens reported include low dose cyclophosphamide with prednisone, CHOP, CEOP and mCOMP [3, 5, 42-44]. Details of these regimens are outlined in tables1-3. Recent data suggest that standard lymphoma-specific chemotherapy is both necessary and effective in PSOT-BL [20, 45]. In two response adapted clinical studies for PTLD, all patients with PSOT-BL required upfront lymphoma specific chemotherapy (R-CHOP in adults and mCOMP in children) due to poor response to RIS and or rituximab alone [3, 20]. A recent report from the French Society of Pediatric Oncology (SFOP) provided preliminary data of 17 pediatric patients with PSOT-BL treated with the intensive LMB (B-NHL specific chemotherapy) with an excellent result [12]. (Table 3)

5.2. Response Based Treatment Strategies

The Ped-PTLD-Pilot-2005 multicenter study of 49 pediatric patients with PTLD used response-adapted sequential immuno-chemotherapy strategy with rituximab +/- chemotherapy in pediatric PTLD (<18 years). If at least a partial response was obtained after 3 weekly doses of rituximab, a further 3 rituximab doses were given every 3 weeks. In the case of stable disease or progression patients received a moderate intensity chemotherapy regimen mCOMP (vincristine, prednisone, cyclophosphamide, and methotrexate) every 4 weeks for 6 cycles. Seven of 49 patients in this study had PSOT-BL. All patients with POST-BL required chemotherapy. Therefore, the protocol was amended to administer mCOMP to all patients with PSOT-BL [3].

In the SFOP study, 17 patients were treated for PSOT-BL. One patient received low-dose cyclophosphamide, steroids and rituximab for very late EBV-negative PSOT-BL but progressed and died of disease despite second-line intensive chemotherapy. The remaining 16 patients were treated according to LMB (intensive BL specific) therapy, 3 after failure of RIS and rituximab monotherapy [12].

Similar data are available from studies in adult patients with PSOT-BL. In the study by Bobillo et al. of 20 adult patients (18 had PSOT-BL and 2 had post hematopoietic stem cell transplant BL), 3 patients received upfront rituximab monotherapy and all required subsequent chemotherapy [45]. In the response adapted study by Zimmerman et al., all patients with PSOT-BL also required R-CHOP chemotherapy, as discussed further below [20].

5.3. Chemotherapy Intensity in PSOT-BL

Intensive chemotherapy regimens are very effective in children and young adults with IC-BL [10, 41, 46-53] and the SFOP data is similarly encouraging for PSOT-BL in children. In this latter study, 16 of 17 children were treated with intensive LMB chemotherapy and there were no treatment related deaths; 14 were long term survivors (median follow up of 9 years). No second malignancies have been observed. The authors concluded that pediatric patients with PSOT-BL can be cured without graft rejection, or unacceptable toxicity [12].

A cooperative group study by Gross et al. of 55 pediatric patients with EBV positive PTLD included 5 patients with Burkitt histology. Patients received a total of 6 cycles of low dose cyclophosphamide in combination with prednisone pulse therapy every 3 weeks with rituximab given once weekly for the first 2 cycles. Four of the 5 patients were long-term disease-free survivors though response data and need for further therapy escalation were not provided [5].

Whether intensive chemotherapy regimens such as LMB therapy [12] are superior to moderate intensity chemotherapy such as mCOMP [3] in PSOT-BL remains to be determined. Because of the small number of patients and the limitations of available data from the SFOP and Ped-PTLD-Pilot-2005 studies, it is not possible to compare the outcome of the 2 regimens used.

A similar question about the necessity of chemotherapy intensity in PSOT-BL was posed by studies in adult patients. The largest study of PSOT-BL in adults provided treatment and outcome data of 20 patients from 10 transplant centers belonging to the GEL/TAMO group. Patients who received CHOP-like regimens attained a CR rate of 73%, while the group who received dose-intensive chemotherapy achieved a CR rate of 83%. Various dose intensive regimens were reported in this study (see Table 1). Patients who received upfront rituximab monotherapy required subsequent chemotherapy. For the whole group 3-year PFS and 3-year OS were 45% [95% CI, 26–64%] and 64% [95% CI, 39–81%] respectively. Two patients (10%) died during treatment due to infection [45].

Zimmermann et al. reported a series of 8 adult patients with PSOT-BL included in the German PTLD registry. Five of the 8 patients received sequential immunochemotherapy consisting of 4 courses of rituximab followed by 4 cycles of CHOP or R-CHOP and all 5 achieved CR. The 2 patients who received first line CHOP and no rituximab were non-responders, both had progression in CNS and died [20]. One advantage of the IC-BL protocols is the incorporation of CNS directed therapy, which may be important in the prevention of CNS relapse in PSOT-BL [54]. Because of the small number of patients reported, the potential role of the sequential treatment strategy in PSOT-BL in adults remains to be determined.

5.4. Cytotoxic T Cell in PTLD and BL

An attractive strategy for the treatment of EBV positive PTLD is based on the use of EBV-specific cytotoxic T lymphocytes (EBV-CTLs). The rationale for exploring T cell therapy for this disease is to restore the underlying immune defect which leads to the development of PTLD without causing bystander organ toxicity and/or further immune suppression [55]. Several studies have demonstrated the promise of this strategy in patients with EBV associated PTLD following hematopoietic and solid organ transplantation [56-59]. A current Children's Oncology Group pilot study, ANHL1522, was designed to study the feasibility of using third-party EBV-CTLs for patients with incomplete response to three cycles of rituximab; there are no preliminary results yet available [60] Currently, the concept of sensitizing BL to EBV-CTLs is being explored [61]. However, experience with PSOT-BL is currently limited, and its role in this subgroup of patients remains to be determined [62].

5.5. CAR-T in PTLD and PSOT-BL

Chimeric antigen receptor T cells (CAR-T) are genetically modified T cells with a chimeric antigen receptor directed against a specific tumor-associated antigen. CAR-T directed against CD19 have shown efficacy in relapsed refractory (r/r) B-ALL and r/r DLBCL, and are FDA approved for these indications [63-67]. The experience for patients with R/R BL is limited to case reports [68-69]. A phase 2 multicenter study is testing CD19 CAR-T in patients ≤25 years old with CD19+ r/r B-NHL in whom one or more therapies have failed, including hematopoietic stem cell transplantation (SCT), (BIANCA, NCT03610724). The study is ongoing, 3 of 8 children enrolled had r/r BL [70]. Concurrent use of immunosuppressive agents was prohibited in most CAR-T trials effectively excluding patients with prior SOT and PTLD. A case series of three adult patients with late PTLD refractory to immunochemotherapy who received CAR-T therapy was concerning for lack of response in spite of all patients developing the acute and expected complications of therapy [71]. This is in contrast to a recent report of successful treatment of PSOT-BL with CD19 CAR-T therapy in a 34-month-old child refractory to rituximab monotherapy. The patient experienced only mild cytokine release syndrome (CRS). He achieved CR and was alive and disease free 16 month after CART infusion [72].

6. Prognostic Factors

Data defining specific prognostic factors for PSOT-BL are extremely limited. In the study of 20 adult patients with PSOT-BL by Bobillo et al., univariate analysis for OS showed only bone marrow infiltration but not age, performance status, stage of disease, time from transplantation to BL, or transplant type, to have an impact [45].

7. Outcome

Standard pediatric protocols in de novo BL consistently utilize intensive multi-agent chemotherapy and more recently immunochemotherapy with excellent outcome [10, 41, 46-49, 73, 74] Despite the intensity of these protocols, treatment related mortality (TRM) is low. In the recent randomized clinical trial investigating the efficacy of adding rituximab to standard LMB chemotherapy, 6 of 328 patients (1.8% of the patients overall) died from toxic effects, four of which were from infections [46]. Patients with PSOT-BL were excluded from this study and prior cooperative group studies in BL [41, 46-48], and data about treatment related mortality in pediatric patients with PSOT-BL are scarce.

In the pediatric study by Cohen-Cogo et al. there was no TRM in patients with PSOT-BL who received intensive LMB-based chemo-immunotherapy. In this cohort of 17 patients with PSOT-BL, all 3 deaths were from progressive disease rather than treatment related toxicity [12].

In another small study 3 of 4 pediatric cases of EBV-driven PSOT-BL, 3 were long term survivors [75].

Another report by Picarsic et al. documented death in 3 of 12 patients with PSOT-BL. One death was treatment related following recurrence, a second was from graft failure and the third died of late complications related to immunosuppression [7].

In adults treated with PSOT-BL intensive chemotherapy regimens have been associated with high TRM [76]. Less intensive therapies, such as R-CHOP, have been better tolerated. There was no treatment-related mortality in a cohort of 5 adult patients treated with R-CHOP or sequential treatment with rituximab followed by CHOP [20]. More recently, Zimmermann et al. reported high TRM (25% of all deaths) in patients with EBV positive PTLD post-SOT who experienced initial treatment failure. Post solid organ transplant Burkitt lymphoma constituted 8.3% of this cohort. Treatment related complications were the leading cause of death [77].

7.1. Potential Long-Term Effects and Need for Therapy Modifications

Long-term follow-up of organ function and late complications of chemotherapy are not described for patients with PSOT-BL. There is no consensus about the ideal regimen and the limitations of therapy modifications in PSOT-BL. When balancing the risks of intensive therapy, it is important to consider that patients with relapsed BL have a dismal outcome [78-80]. Therefore, treatment reductions have to be considered with caution.

Table 1. POST-BL treatment in adults, case series

Ref.	Organ	# BL	Gender	Age at BL, median (range in years)	Time to BL, median (range in years)	RIS	Treatment regimens	Treatment response	Survival (in years)
[20]	Heart (1) Liver (3) Kidney (3) Kidney, pancreas (1)	8	7M/1F	38 (18-54)	5.7 (0.2- 12.5)	5	5: Sequential immuno-chemotherapy (R, R-CHOP) 2: CHOP 1: Cy followed by sequential therapy	Sequential therapy: 5 CR, 1 relapsed Frontline CHOP: 2 No response	CR (median 7.7, range 0.2-16) OS (3.1) TRM: None
[23]	Heart (2) Liver (2) Kidney (1)	5	5M/0F	65 (44 -70)	4.8 (2.9-5.5)	NR	4: R-CHOP 1: R	4: CR 1: PR	1: CR (8.5) 4: Dead of unrelated causes (0.3-0.9)
[45]	Heart (2) Liver (3) Kidney (11) Lung(2) HSCT (2)	20	9M/11F	45 (23–71)	7.2 (0.2–21.7)	All	9: R-CHOP 3: Burkimab regimen 3: rituximab monotherapy 1: CHOP 2: LLA/LB97 1: CODOX-M/IVAC 1: R-EPOCH	15: CR CHOP like: CR 8 of 11 Intensive regimens: CR 5 of 6 Rituximab monotherapy: CR 2 of 3: (all relapsed) 8: Relapse 2 DOC (1 R-CHOP 1 CHOP)	Median PFS (1.3) Median OS (11.4) 3-year PFS 45% 3-year OS 64%

Table 1. (Continued)

Ref.	Organ	# BL	Gender	Age at BL, median (range in years)	Time to BL, median (range in years)	RIS	Treatment regimens	Treatment response	Survival (in years)
[76]	Heart (1) Liver (1) Kidney (2) HSCT (1)	5	3M/2F	54 (20-66)	0.2-12.0	All	PETHEMA ALL3/97 protocol	3:CR (0.4-1.4) 2:DOC	2: CR: (0.5, 1.4) 3: DOC (0.1-0.2)

PSOT-BL: post-solid organ transplant Burkitt lymphoma; M: male, F: female; DOC: Death of treatment complications; RIS: reduction of immune suppression; BL: Burkitt lymphoma; R: complete remission; NR: not reported, TRM: treatment related mortality; HSCT: Hematopoietic stem cell transplantation.

[20] Cy: cyclophosphamide; Sequential immunochemotehrapy: 4 courses of rituximab (R) followed by 4 cycles of CHOP (cyclophosphamide, doxorubicin, vincristine, and prednisolone) or R plus CHOP (R-CHOP); CHOP: cyclophosphamide 750 mg/m2 on day 1, doxorubicin 50 mg/m2 on day 1, vincristine 1.4 mg/m2 (maximum, 2 mg) on day 1, and prednisolone 100 mg on days 1 through 5 every 22 days; cyclophosphamide; R-CHOP:CHOP plus rituximab 375 mg/m2 on day 1 every 8 days; and Ara-C/MTX IT consisted of Ara-C 40 mg IT and MTX 15 mg IT.

[45] Burkimab regimen: rituximab and high-dose chemotherapy including high-dose methotrexate (MTX) and Ara-C; LLA/LB97: protocol details not specified; CODOX-M/IVAC: cyclophosphamide, vincristine, doxorubicin, high-dose methotrexate/ifosfamide, etoposide, high-dose cytarabine (number of cycles not specified); R-EPOCH: rituximab, etoposide prednisone, vincristine, cyclophosphamide, doxorubicin (number of cycles not specified).

[76] The PETHEMA ALL3/97 regimen: prophase: Prednisone 60 mg/m2 for 5 days, cyclophosphamide 200 mg/m2; cycle A (ifosfamide 800 mg/m2 iv and dexamethasone 10 mg/m2 iv on days 1–5, vincristine 2mg iv, methotrexate 3 g/m2 iv on day 1, etoposide 100 mg/m2 iv on days 4 and 5 and cytarabine 150 mg/m2 iv every 12 h on days 4 and 5; cycle B (cyclophosphamide 200 mg/m2 iv and dexamethasone 10 mg/m2 days 1–5, vincristine 2mg, methotrexate 3 g/m2 on day 1, doxorubicin 25 mg/m2 days 4 and 5), alternating every 3 weeks with cycle A for a total number of 5 consolidation cycles (total duration of therapy: 18 weeks). CNS prophylaxis consisted of 12 doses of methotrexate (12 mg), cytarabine (30 mg) and hydrocortisone (20 mg).

Table 2. Individual adult case reports of PSOT-BL

Ref	Organ	Age† /gender	Time to BL††	Site	RIS	Treatment regimen	Last f/u alive in CR (in Years)
[26]	Heart	54 M	3	bowel, mesentery, LN, mediastinum	Yes	PACE-BOM, IT	CR (4)
[31]	Kidney	45 F	8	abdominal mass, mesentery	Yes	Cy, ASCT	Died of second PTLD (0.2)
[32]	Kidney	43 F	2.5	LN, liver,	yes	CODOX-M/IVAC	NR
[33]	Liver	44 M	4	abdominal mass	NR	NR	NR
[62]*	NR	NR	NR	NR	Yes	3 patients: 1: R (refractory) 1: CT (NOS): NR 1:CTLs	DOD
[81]	Heart	24 F	6	pelvis	Yes	R-CEOP	CR(1.6)
[82]	Kidney, pancreas	39 M	7	abdominal/pelvic mass, mandible, LN	Yes	HD-MTX, R, D, O, IT	CR (2)
[83]	kidney	46 M	12	stomach	Yes	NR	DOC (0.1)
[84]	Kidney	55 F	8	breast	Yes	6-cycles hyper-CVAD with IT, alternating with HD-MTX, HD ARAC	CR (4)
[85]	Liver	63 M	1.5	bone marrow	Yes	8-cycles hyper-CVAD alternating with HD-MTX, HD ARAC	CR (NR)

† Age in years at Diagnosis of PSOT-BL; ††time from Transplant to BL; *3 patients; PSOT-BL: post-solid organ transplant Burkitt lymphoma; CR: complete remission; RIS: DOD: dead of disease; f/u: follow up; LN: Lymph Nodes; NR: Not reported; CT: chemotherapy; NOS: not otherwise specified); Cy: cyclophosphamide; D; doxorubicin; HD-MTX: high-dose methotrexate; CTLs: cytotoxic T cells, R-CEOP: R: rituximab; C: cyclophosphamide; O: vincristine, E: etoposide, P: prednisone; PACE-BOM: prednisolone, doxorubicin, cyclophosphamide, etoposide, alternating with bleomycin, vincristine, melphalan for 12 cycles and intrathecal methotrexate alternating with cytarabine twice weekly for 3 weeks, then once weekly for 16 doses total; IT: intrathecal chemotherapy; hyper-CVAD: cyclophosphamide, vincristine, doxorubicin, dexamethasone), HD ARAC: high dose cytarabine; ASCT: autologous Stem cell transplantation; CODOX-M/IVAC cyclophosphamide, vincristine, doxorubicin and methotrexate, alternating with etoposide, ifosfamide and cytarabine.

Table 3. POST-BL treatment in children, case series and case reports

[Ref]	Organ	# BL	Gender	Age at BL Median (range)**	Time to BL Median (range)**	IST	Treatment regimens	Outcome (duration of CR in years)
Case series								
[3]*	NR	7	NR	NR	NR	NR	6: mCOMP 1: NR	4: CR
[5]*	NR	5	NR	NR	NR	NR	R, P, Low dose Cy	4: CR 1: DOD
[7]	Heart (5) Liver (5) Small intestine (1) Kidney (1)	12	9 M/3F	3 (0.2-16.3	4.3 (0.5-8.9)	NR	7: various regimens 5: NA	9: CR (median: 7.7, range: 0.2-16) 3 Deaths: 1 DOC 1 Graft failure 1 Infection
[12]	Liver: (11) Kidney (5) Liver-kidney (1)	17	12M/5F	6.9 (2.6-15.6)	3.4 (1.3-13.0)	RIS: 16	16: LMB regimen (3 after failure of R) 1: R, Low dose Cy Modifications: 7: reduced HD-MTX 8: rituximab	14 CR (median 9, range NR) 1 DOD 2 early deaths 2^{ry} to tumor lysis TRM: None
[75]	Heart (4)	4	3M/1F	(9-17.5)	(2-5.5)	CIS:1 RIS: 3	1: multiple regimens 3: UKCCSG protocol NHL 9001	3 CR (1.9, 3.5, 8) 1 DOC
Case reports								
[Ref]	Organ	# BL	Age/gender	Age at BL (in years)	Time to BL (in years)	IS	Treatment regimens	Outcome (duration of CR in years)
[23]	Kidney (1)	2	16 M	16	1.1	NR	R-CHOP	CR (2.8)

[Ref]	Organ	# BL	Gender	Age at BL Median (range)**	Time to BL Median (range)**	IST	Treatment regimens	Outcome (duration of CR in years)
	Liver (1)		15 M	15	0.9		Intensive CT (NOS)	CR (6.6)
[33]	Liver (1)	1	11 M	11	5.0	CIS	R	DOC (0.5)
[72]	Liver (1)	1	2.8 M	2.8	1.8	CIS	R, CT (NOS), resection CD19 CAR-T after progression	CR (1.3)
[86]	Liver (1)	1	3.5 M	3.5	2.1	RIS	etoposide, doxorubicin, cyclophosphamide, corticosteroids, IT	CR (6.3)

PSOT-BL: post-solid organ transplant Burkitt lymphoma; *Patients characteristics specific to patients with Burkitt lymphoma subtype where not reported; BL: **in years; Burkitt lymphoma; CR: complete remission; NR: not reported, CT: chemotherapy; NOS: Not otherwise specified; M: male, F: female; DOD: died of disease (BL); DOC: death of treatment complications; TRM: treatment related mortality; IST: immunosuppressive therapy; RIS: reduction of immune suppression; CIS; cessation of immune suppression; Cy; cyclophosphamide; HD-MTX: high dose methotrexate; R-mCOMP; Rituximab 375 mg/m2 IV weekly × 3 doses, If CR or PR (32): Rituximab 375 mg/m2 IV × 3 doses If SD or PD: vincristine on day 1, prednisone on day 1, cyclophosphamide on day 1, methotrexate on day 15 × 6 cycles; R, P, Cy low: rituximab, prednisone, low dose cyclophosphamide; R-CHOP: R-CHOP: rituximab 375 mg/m2 on day 1, cyclophosphamide 750 mg/m2 on day 1, doxorubicin 50 mg/m2 on day 1; vincristine 1.4 mg/m2 (maximum, 2 mg) on day 1, and prednisolone 100 mg on days 1-5 every 22 days; rituximab 375 mg/m2 every 8 days.

8. Organ Specific Treatment Considerations

8.1. Cardiac

Doxorubicin is a component of chemotherapy regimens in both pediatric and adult IC-BL. However its long-term effects of its administration in heart transplant recipients has not been studied.

Two small pediatric case series describing cardiac transplant recipients diagnosed with PSOT-BL are available [7, 75]. Of the 4 cases reported by Windebank et al., 3 were long term survivors. All 4 patients received doxorubicin without dose modification and one received dexrazoxane. Anthracycline related cardiac toxicity did not occur. However, 2 patients experienced cardiac allograft vasculopathy; one died before receiving a second transplant and the other successfully underwent a second transplant [75]. Among 12 children with PSOT-BL reported by Picarsic et al., 5 were cardiac transplant recipients. Therapy was described in 4 of these 5 patients and included doxorubicin. Three of the 12 children in this study died. One of these three was a cardiac transplant recipient who died of therapy-related complications (sepsis and multiorgan failure) one month from diagnosis of PSOT-BL. At autopsy, there was no evidence of residual BL [7].

AbdelHameid et al. recently reported a case of PSOT-BL post-heart transplant in a young adult where a non-anthracycline containing chemotherapy regimen was chosen specifically to avoid cardiotoxicity. The patient received 6 cycles of R-COEP (rituximab, cyclophosphamide, vincristine, etoposide, prednisone) over 6 months followed by 3 cycles of high-dose methotrexate (MTX) over 3 months for CNS prophylaxis. The patient was in CR 19 months post-treatment. They proposed that an anthracycline-free regimen could be an option for patients with PSOT-BL after heart transplantation [81].

Additional case series and reports in adults and children are reported in Tables 1-3.

8.2. Renal and Hepatic Toxicity

High dose methotrexate is a component of therapy in the majority of pediatric regimens for IC-BL. This component of therapy constitutes a challenge for renal transplant and potentially liver transplant recipients. In the study by Cohen-Gogo et al., 4 of 17 patients required dialysis/ hemofiltration at diagnosis of PSOT-BL and 7 had reduction of the methotrexate dosing. No further specifics were provided about the indication and the level of dose reduction, or the organ transplanted [12]. In a study of 4 pediatric patients with PSOT -BL, methotrexate was omitted in one patient and delayed in another, both patients were long term survivors [75]. These cases provide some evidence that modifications of these intensive pediatric regimens may be necessary. The effect of these treatment reductions on lymphoma free survival and overall survival remains to be determined. Of special interest is investigation of the role of the addition of rituximab in allowing treatment reductions without adversely affecting outcome.

Conclusion and Perspectives

The small number of patients who develop PSOT-BL, and their exclusion from past studies of IC-BL and some studies of PTLD, add to the challenge of advancing the knowledge of clinical and pathologic characteristics, optimal treatment regimens and outcome. Based on available data, successful treatment of young patients with PSOT-BL with full BL therapy is possible, although some treatment modifications for individual patients may be necessary. On the other hand, reports of durable complete remissions with less intensive therapy provide the rationale for identifying patients who can be successfully treated with less intensive therapy. Integrating details of treatment administered, disease response, and toxicities in large registries will be an important step in designing therapies specific for this small but challenging subgroup of patients. Inclusion of patients in prospective international studies can provide important data particularly for short and long-term toxicities and graft outcome to inform guidelines for treatment modifications based on the organ transplanted. Finally studying the genomics of PSOT-BL compared to IC-BL could provide new understanding of differences in disease biology and discovery of new targeted treatment approaches.

Acknowledgements

The authors wish to thank Dr. Denis Miller for reviewing this chapter.

References

[1] Mbulaiteye, S. M., C. A. Clarke, L. M. Morton, T. M. Gibson, K. Pawlish, D. D. Weisenburger, C. F. Lynch, M. T. Goodman, and E. A. Engels. 2013. "Burkitt lymphoma risk in U.S. solid organ transplant recipients." *Am J Hematol* 88 (4):245-50. doi: 10.1002/ajh.23385.

[2] Yanik, E. L., M. S. Shiels, J. M. Smith, C. A. Clarke, C. F. Lynch, A. R. Kahn, L. Koch, K. S. Pawlish, and E. A. Engels. 2017. "Contribution of solid organ transplant recipients to the pediatric non-hodgkin lymphoma burden in the United States." *Cancer* 123 (23):4663-4671. doi: 10.1002/cncr.30923.

[3] Maecker-Kolhoff, B., R. Beier, M. Zimmermann, B. Schlegelberger, U. Baumann, C. Mueller, L. Pape, A. Reiter, C. Rossig, S. Schubert, B. Toenshoff, A. Wingen, B. Meissner, C. Kebelmann-Betzing, G. Henze, H. H. Kreipe, and C. Klein. 2014 "Response-adapted sequential Immuno-chemotherapy of post-Transplant lymphoproliferative disorders in pediatric solid Organ Transplant recipients: results from the prospective Ped-PTLD 2005 trial". *Blood* 124:4468.

[4] Kanzelmeyer, N. K., B. Maecker-Kolhoff, H. Zierhut, C. Lerch, M. Verboom, D. Haffner, and L. Pape. 2018. "Graft outcomes following

diagnosis of post-transplant lymphoproliferative disease in pediatric kidney recipients: a retrospective study." *Transpl Int* 31 (4):367-376. doi: 10.1111/tri.13071.

[5] Gross, T. G., M. A. Orjuela, S. L. Perkins, J. R. Park, J. C. Lynch, M. S. Cairo, L. M. Smith, and R. J. Hayashi. 2012. "Low-dose chemotherapy and rituximab for posttransplant lymphoproliferative disease (PTLD): a Children's Oncology Group Report." *Am J Transplant* 12 (11):3069-75. doi: 10.1111/j.1600-6143.2012. 04206.x.

[6] Schober, T., T. Framke, H. Kreipe, T. F. Schulz, A. Grosshennig, K. Hussein, U. Baumann, L. Pape, S. Schubert, A. M. Wingen, T. Jack, A. Koch, C. Klein, and B. Maecker-Kolhoff. 2013. "Characteristics of early and late PTLD development in pediatric solid organ transplant recipients." *Transplantation* 95 (1):240-6. doi: 10.1097/TP.0b013e318277e344.

[7] Picarsic, J., R. Jaffe, G. Mazariegos, S. A. Webber, D. Ellis, M. D. Green, and M. Reyes-Mugica. 2011. "Post-Transplant Burkitt Lymphoma Is a More Aggressive and Distinct Form of Post-Transplant Lymphoproliferative Disorder." *Cancer* 117 (19): 4540-50 https://doi.org/10.1002/cncr.26001.

[8] Thacker, Nirav, and Oussama Abla. 2019. "Epidemiology of Non-Hodgkin Lymphomas in Childhood and Adolescence." In *Non-Hodgkin's Lymphoma in Childhood and Adolescence*, 15-22.

[9] Clarke, C. A., L. M. Morton, C. Lynch, R. M. Pfeiffer, E. C. Hall, T. M. Gibson, D. D. Weisenburger, O. Martinez-Maza, S. K. Hussain, J. Yang, E. T. Chang, and E. A. Engels. 2013. "Risk of lymphoma subtypes after solid organ transplantation in the United States." *Br J Cancer* 109 (1):280-8. doi: 10.1038/bjc.2013.294.

[10] Egan, Grace, Weitzman, Sheila, and Alexander, Sarah. 2019. "Burkitt Lymphoma and Diffuse Large B-Cell Lymphoma." In *Non-Hodgkin's Lymphoma in Childhood and Adolescence*, 167-183l

[11] Burkhardt, B., M. Zimmermann, I. Oschlies, F. Niggli, G. Mann, R. Parwaresch, H. Riehm, M. Schrappe, A. Reiter, and B. F. M. Group. 2005. "The impact of age and gender on biology, clinical features

and treatment outcome of non-Hodgkin lymphoma in childhood and adolescence." *Br J Haematol* 131 (1):39-49. doi: 10.1111/j.1365-2141.2005.05735.x.

[12] Cohen-Gogo, S., J. Landman-Parker, G. Michel, H. Pacquement, J. Michon, Y. Bertrand, B. Nelken, C. Schmitt, N. Mahlaoui, C. Briandett, A. Jourdain, P. Lutz, J. Clavel, T. Molina, T. Leblanc, D. Habes, E. Jacuemin, R. Salomon, V. Minard-Colin and C. Patte. "LMB chemotherapy is effective for Burkitt Lymphoma occurring after sold organ transplantation in children: A report from the societe francaise des cancers de L'enfante (SFCE)." In: The 51st Congress of the International Society of Paediatric Oncology (SIOP) Lyon, France, October 23-26, 2019. *Pediatr Blood Cancer*. 2019;66 Suppl 4:e27989. doi:10.1002/pbc.27989.

[13] Mynarek, M., T. Schober, U. Behrends, and B. Maecker-Kolhoff. 2013. "Posttransplant lymphoproliferative disease after pediatric solid organ transplantation." *Clin Dev Immunol* 2013:814973. doi: 10.1155/2013/814973.

[14] Swerdlow, S. H., E. Campo, S. A. Pileri, N. L. Harris, H. Stein, R. Siebert, R. Advani, M. Ghielmini, G. A. Salles, A. D. Zelenetz, and E. S. Jaffe. 2016. "The 2016 revision of the World Health Organization classification of lymphoid neoplasms." *Blood* 127 (20):2375-90. doi: 10.1182/blood-2016-01-643569.

[15] Dalla-Favera, R., M. Bregni, J. Erikson, D. Patterson, R. C. Gallo, and C. M. Croce. 1982. "Human c-myc onc gene is located on the region of chromosome 8 that is translocated in Burkitt lymphoma cells." *Proc Natl Acad Sci USA* 79 (24):7824-7. doi: 10.1073/pnas.79.24.7824.

[16] Klein, G. 1983. "Specific chromosomal translocations and the genesis of B-cell-derived tumors in mice and men." *Cell* 32 (2):311-5. doi: 10.1016/0092-8674(83)90449-x.

[17] Klapproth, K., and T. Wirth. 2010. "Advances in the understanding of MYC-induced lymphomagenesis." *Br J Haematol* 149 (4):484-97. doi: 10.1111/j.1365-2141.2010.08159.x.

[18] Magrath, I. 2012. "Epidemiology: clues to the pathogenesis of Burkitt lymphoma." *Br J Haematol* 156 (6):744-56. doi: 10.1111/j. 1365-2141.2011.09013.x.

[19] Gong, J. Z., T. T. Stenzel, E. R. Bennett, A. S. Lagoo, C. H. Dunphy, J. O. Moore, D. A. Rizzieri, J. H. Tepperberg, P. Papenhausen, and P. J. Buckley. 2003. "Burkitt lymphoma arising in organ transplant recipients: a clinicopathologic study of five cases." *Am J Surg Pathol* 27 (6):818-27. doi: 10.1097/00000478-200306000-00014.

[20] Zimmermann, H., Reinke, P., Neuhaus, R., Lehmkuhl, H., Oertel, S., Atta, J., Planker, M., Gartner, B., Lenze, D., Anagnostopoulos, I., Riess, H., and Trappe, R. U. 2012. "Burkitt post-transplantation lymphoma in adult solid organ transplant recipients: sequential immunochemotherapy with rituximab (R) followed by cyclophosphamide, doxorubicin, vincristine, and prednisone (CHOP) or R-CHOP is safe and effective in an analysis of 8 patients." *Cancer* 118 (19):4715-24. doi: 10.1002/cncr.27482.

[21] Piccaluga, P. P., G. De Falco, M. Kustagi, A. Gazzola, C. Agostinelli, C. Tripodo, E. Leucci, A. Onnis, A. Astolfi, M. R. Sapienza, C. Bellan, S. Lazzi, L. Tumwine, M. Mawanda, M. Ogwang, V. Calbi, S. Formica, A. Califano, S. A. Pileri, and L. Leoncini. 2011. "Gene expression analysis uncovers similarity and differences among Burkitt lymphoma subtypes." *Blood* 117 (13):3596-608. doi: 10.1182/blood-2010-08-301556.

[22] Salaverria, I., I. Martin-Guerrero, R. Wagener, M. Kreuz, C. W. Kohler, J. Richter, B. Pienkowska-Grela, P. Adam, B. Burkhardt, A. Claviez, C. Damm-Welk, H. G. Drexler, M. Hummel, E. S. Jaffe, R. Kuppers, C. Lefebvre, J. Lisfeld, M. Loffler, R. A. Macleod, I. Nagel, I. Oschlies, M. Rosolowski, R. B. Russell, G. Rymkiewicz, D. Schindler, M. Schlesner, R. Scholtysik, C. Schwaenen, R. Spang, M. Szczepanowski, L. Trumper, I. Vater, S. Wessendorf, W. Klapper, R. Siebert, Project Molecular Mechanisms in Malignant Lymphoma Network, and Group Berlin-Frankfurt-Munster Non-Hodgkin Lymphoma. 2014. "A recurrent 11q aberration pattern characterizes a subset of MYC-negative high-grade B-cell

lymphomas resembling Burkitt lymphoma." *Blood* 123 (8):1187-98. doi: 10.1182/blood-2013-06-507996.

[23] Ferreiro, J. F., J. Morscio, D. Dierickx, L. Marcelis, G. Verhoef, P. Vandenberghe, T. Tousseyn, and I. Wlodarska. 2015. "Post-transplant molecularly defined Burkitt lymphomas are frequently MYC-negative and characterized by the 11q-gain/loss pattern." *Haematologica* 100 (7):e275-9. doi: 10.3324/haematol.2015.124305.

[24] Everly, M. J., R. D. Bloom, D. E. Tsai, and J. Trofe. 2007. "Post-transplant lymphoproliferative disorder." *Ann Pharmacother* 41 (11):1850-8. doi: 10.1345/aph.1G706.

[25] Shroff, R., and L. Rees. 2004. "The post-transplant lymphoproliferative disorder-a literature review." *Pediatr Nephrol* 19 (4):369-77. doi: 10.1007/s00467-003-1392-x.

[26] Hunt, B. J., J. A. Thomas, M. Burke, H. Walker, M. Yacoub, and D. H. Crawford. 1996. "Epstein-Barr virus associated Burkitt lymphoma in a heart transplant recipient." *Transplantation* 62 (6):869-72. doi: 10.1097/00007890-199609270-00030.

[27] Srivatsa, Kavitha, and Mary Taj. 2021. "Childhood post-transplant lymphoproliferative disorder." *Paediatrics and Child Health* 31 (3):95-101. doi: 10.1016/j.paed.2020.12.001.

[28] Morscio, J., D. Dierickx, and T. Tousseyn. 2013. "Molecular pathogenesis of B-cell posttransplant lymphoproliferative disorder: what do we know so far?" *Clin Dev Immunol* 2013:150835. doi: 10.1155/2013/150835.

[29] Riches, J., K. Naresh, A. Reid, and D. Macdonald. 2009. "Burkitt lymphoma following renal transplantation." *Br J Haematol* 146 (6):583. doi: 10.1111/j.1365-2141.2009.07583.x.

[30] Johnson, L. R., M. A. Nalesnik, and S. H. Swerdlow. 2006. "Impact of Epstein-Barr virus in monomorphic B-cell posttransplant lymphoproliferative disorders: a histogenetic study." *Am J Surg Pathol* 30 (12):1604-12. doi: 10.1097/01.pas.0000213317.59176.d2.

[31] Lohrisch, C. A., T. J. Nevill, M. J. Barnett, D. E. Hogge, J. M. Connors, P. A. Keown, and R. D. Gascoyne. 2000. "Development of a biologically distinct EBV-related lymphoproliferative disorder

following autologous bone marrow transplantation for an EBV-negative post-renal allograft Burkitt's lymphoma." *Leuk Lymphoma* 39 (1-2):195-201. doi: 10.3109/10428190009053554.

[32] Harris, E., S. Paneesha, N. Jackson, L. Jones, and P. Mahendra. 2002. "Burkitt's lymphoma: single-centre experience with modified BFM protocol." *Clin Lab Haematol* 24 (2):111-4. doi: 10.1046/j.1365-2257.2002.00429.x.

[33] Pasquale M. A., D. Weppler, J. Smith, M. Icardi, A. Amador, M. Gonzalez, T. Kato, A. Tzakis, and P. Ruiz. 2002. "Burkitt's lymphoma variant of post-transplant lymphoproliferative disease (PTLD)." *Pathology & Oncology Research* 8 (2):105-108. doi: 10.1007/bf03033718.

[34] Nelson, B. P., M. A. Nalesnik, D. W. Bahler, J. Locker, J. J. Fung, and S. H. Swerdlow. 2000. "Epstein-Barr virus-negative post-transplant lymphoproliferative disorders: a distinct entity?" *Am J Surg Pathol* 24 (3):375-85. doi: 10.1097/00000478-200003000-00006.

[35] Thorley-Lawson, D. A., and A. Gross. 2004. "Persistence of the Epstein-Barr virus and the origins of associated lymphomas." *N Engl J Med* 350 (13):1328-37. doi: 10.1056/NEJMra032015.

[36] San-Juan, R., P. Comoli, S. Caillard, B. Moulin, H. H. Hirsch, P. Meylan, and Escmid Study Group of Infection in Compromised Hosts. 2014. "Epstein-Barr virus-related post-transplant lymphoproliferative disorder in solid organ transplant recipients." *Clin Microbiol Infect* 20 Suppl 7:109-18. doi: 10.1111/1469-0691.12534.

[37] Funk, G. A., R. Gosert, and H. H. Hirsch. 2007. "Viral dynamics in transplant patients: implications for disease." *Lancet Infect Dis* 7 (7):460-72. doi: 10.1016/S1473-3099(07)70159-7.

[38] Cockfield, S. M. 2001. "Identifying the patient at risk for post-transplant lymphoproliferative disorder." *Transpl Infect Dis* 3 (2):70-8. doi: 10.1034/j.1399-3062.2001.003002070.x

[39] Gartner, B., and J. K. Preiksaitis. 2010. "EBV viral load detection in clinical virology." *J Clin Virol* 48 (2):82-90. doi: 10.1016/j.jcv.2010.03.016.

[40] Allen, U. D., J. K. Preiksaitis, and A. S. T. Infectious Diseases Community of Practice. 2013. "Epstein-Barr virus and posttransplant lymphoproliferative disorder in solid organ transplantation." *Am J Transplant* 13 Suppl 4:107-20. doi: 10.1111/ajt.12104.

[41] Cairo, M. S., R. Sposto, M. Gerrard, A. Auperin, S. C. Goldman, L. Harrison, R. Pinkerton, M. Raphael, K. McCarthy, S. L. Perkins, and C. Patte. 2012. "Advanced stage, increased lactate dehydrogenase, and primary site, but not adolescent age (>/= 15 years), are associated with an increased risk of treatment failure in children and adolescents with mature B-cell non-Hodgkin's lymphoma: results of the FAB LMB 96 study." *J Clin Oncol* 30 (4):387-93. doi: 10.1200/JCO.2010.33.3369.

[42] Trappe, R. U., D. Dierickx, H. Zimmermann, F. Morschhauser, P. Mollee, J. M. Zaucha, M. H. Dreyling, U. Duhrsen, P. Reinke, G. Verhoef, M. Subklewe, A. Huttmann, T. Tousseyn, G. Salles, V. Kliem, I. A. Hauser, C. Tarella, E. Van Den Neste, O. Gheysens, I. Anagnostopoulos, V. Leblond, H. Riess, and S. Choquet. 2017. "Response to Rituximab Induction Is a Predictive Marker in B-Cell Post-Transplant Lymphoproliferative Disorder and Allows Successful Stratification Into Rituximab or R-CHOP Consolidation in an International, Prospective, Multicenter Phase II Trial." *J Clin Oncol* 35 (5):536-543. doi: 10.1200/JCO.2016.69.3564.

[43] Trappe, R., S. Oertel, V. Leblond, P. Mollee, M. Sender, P. Reinke, R. Neuhaus, H. Lehmkuhl, H. A. Horst, G. Salles, F. Morschhauser, A. Jaccard, T. Lamy, M. Leithauser, H. Zimmermann, I. Anagnostopoulos, M. Raphael, H. Riess, S. Choquet, PTLD Study Group German, and PTLD Network European. 2012. "Sequential treatment with rituximab followed by CHOP chemotherapy in adult B-cell post-transplant lymphoproliferative disorder (PTLD): the prospective international multicentre phase 2 PTLD-1 trial." *Lancet Oncol* 13 (2):196-206. doi: 10.1016/S1470-2045(11)70300-X.

[44] Zimmermann, H., and R. U. Trappe. 2013. "EBV and posttransplantation lymphoproliferative disease: what to do?" Hematology, *Am*

Soc Hematol Educ Program 2013:95-102. doi: 10.1182/asheducation-2013.1.95.

[45] Bobillo, S., P. Abrisqueta, B. Sanchez-Gonzalez, E. Gine, S. Romero, M. Alcoceba, E. Gonzalez-Barca, S. Gonzalez de Villambrosia, J. M. Sancho, P. Gomez, L. Bento, J. Montoro, S. Montes, A. Lopez, F. Bosch, and Osea Grupo Espanol de Linfomas/Trasplante Autologo de Medula. 2018. "Posttransplant monomorphic Burkitt's lymphoma: clinical characteristics and outcome of a multicenter series." *Ann Hematol* 97 (12):2417-2424. doi: 10.1007/s00277-018-3473-8.

[46] Minard-Colin, V., A. Auperin, M. Pillon, G. A. A. Burke, D. A. Barkauskas, K. Wheatley, R. F. Delgado, S. Alexander, A. Uyttebroeck, C. M. Bollard, J. Zsiros, M. Csoka, B. Kazanowska, A. K. Chiang, R. R. Miles, A. Wotherspoon, P. C. Adamson, G. Vassal, C. Patte, T. G. Gross, Lymphoma European Intergroup for Childhood Non-Hodgkin, and Group Children's Oncology. 2020. "Rituximab for High-Risk, Mature B-Cell Non-Hodgkin's Lymphoma in Children." *N Engl J Med* 382 (23):2207-2219. doi: 10.1056/NEJMoa1915315.

[47] Cairo, M. S., M. Gerrard, R. Sposto, A. Auperin, C. R. Pinkerton, J. Michon, C. Weston, S. L. Perkins, M. Raphael, K. McCarthy, C. Patte, and Fab LMB International Study Committee. 2007. "Results of a randomized international study of high-risk central nervous system B non-Hodgkin lymphoma and B acute lymphoblastic leukemia in children and adolescents." *Blood* 109 (7):2736-43. doi: 10.1182/blood-2006-07-036665.

[48] Patte, C., A. Auperin, M. Gerrard, J. Michon, R. Pinkerton, R. Sposto, C. Weston, M. Raphael, S. L. Perkins, K. McCarthy, M. S. Cairo, and Fab LMB International Study Committee. 2007. "Results of the randomized international FAB/LMB96 trial for intermediate risk B-cell non-Hodgkin lymphoma in children and adolescents: it is possible to reduce treatment for the early responding patients." *Blood* 109 (7):2773-80. doi: 10.1182/blood-2006-07-036673.

[49] Woessmann, W., K. Seidemann, G. Mann, M. Zimmermann, B. Burkhardt, I. Oschlies, W. D. Ludwig, T. Klingebiel, N. Graf, B. Gruhn, H. Juergens, F. Niggli, R. Parwaresch, H. Gadner, H. Riehm, M. Schrappe, A. Reiter, and B. F. M. Group. 2005. "The impact of the methotrexate administration schedule and dose in the treatment of children and adolescents with B-cell neoplasms: a report of the BFM Group Study NHL-BFM95." *Blood* 105 (3):948-58. doi: 10.1182/blood-2004-03-0973.

[50] Jacobson, C., and A. LaCasce. 2014. "How I treat Burkitt lymphoma in adults." *Blood* 124 (19):2913-20. doi: 10.1182/blood-2014-06-538504.

[51] Noy, A., J. Y. Lee, E. Cesarman, R. Ambinder, R. Baiocchi, E. Reid, L. Ratner, N. Wagner-Johnston, L. Kaplan, and Aids Malignancy Consortium. 2015. "AMC 048: modified CODOX-M/IVAC-rituximab is safe and effective for HIV-associated Burkitt lymphoma." *Blood* 126 (2):160-6. doi: 10.1182/blood-2015-01-623900.

[52] Roschewski, M., K. Dunleavy, J. S. Abramson, B. L. Powell, B. K. Link, P. Patel, P. J. Bierman, D. Jagadeesh, R. T. Mitsuyasu, D. Peace, P. R. Watson, W. T. Hanna, C. Melani, A. N. Lucas, S. M. Steinberg, S. Pittaluga, E. S. Jaffe, J. W. Friedberg, B. S. Kahl, R. F. Little, N. L. Bartlett, M. A. Fanale, A. Noy, and W. H. Wilson. 2020. "Multicenter Study of Risk-Adapted Therapy with Dose-Adjusted EPOCH-R in Adults with Untreated Burkitt Lymphoma." *J Clin Oncol* 38 (22):2519-2529. doi: 10.1200/JCO.20.00303.

[53] Dunleavy, Kieron, Stefania Pittaluga, Margaret Shovlin, Seth M. Steinberg, Diane Cole, Cliona Grant, Brigitte Widemann, Louis M. Staudt, Elaine S. Jaffe, Richard F. Little, and Wyndham H. Wilson. 2013. "Low-Intensity Therapy in Adults with Burkitt's Lymphoma." *New England Journal of Medicine* 369 (20):1915-1925. doi: 10.1056/nejmoa1308392.

[54] Dierickx, D., T. Tousseyn, and O. Gheysens. 2015. "How I treat posttransplant lymphoproliferative disorders." *Blood* 126 (20):2274-83. doi: 10.1182/blood-2015-05-615872.

[55] Bollard, C. M., C. M. Rooney, and H. E. Heslop. 2012. "T-cell therapy in the treatment of post-transplant lymphoproliferative disease." *Nat Rev Clin Oncol* 9 (9):510-9. doi: 10.1038/nrclinonc.2012.111.

[56] Heslop, H. E., K. S. Slobod, M. A. Pule, G. A. Hale, A. Rousseau, C. A. Smith, C. M. Bollard, H. Liu, M. F. Wu, R. J. Rochester, P. J. Amrolia, J. L. Hurwitz, M. K. Brenner, and C. M. Rooney. 2010. "Long-term outcome of EBV-specific T-cell infusions to prevent or treat EBV-related lymphoproliferative disease in transplant recipients." *Blood* 115 (5):925-35. doi: 10.1182/blood-2009-08-239186.

[57] Doubrovina, E., B. Oflaz-Sozmen, S. E. Prockop, N. A. Kernan, S. Abramson, J. Teruya-Feldstein, C. Hedvat, J. F. Chou, G. Heller, J. N. Barker, F. Boulad, H. Castro-Malaspina, D. George, A. Jakubowski, G. Koehne, E. B. Papadopoulos, A. Scaradavou, T. N. Small, R. Khalaf, J. W. Young, and R. J. O'Reilly. 2012. "Adoptive immunotherapy with unselected or EBV-specific T cells for biopsy-proven EBV+ lymphomas after allogeneic hematopoietic cell transplantation." *Blood* 119 (11):2644-56. doi: 10.1182/blood-2011-08-371971.

[58] Haque, T., G. M. Wilkie, M. M. Jones, C. D. Higgins, G. Urquhart, P. Wingate, D. Burns, K. McAulay, M. Turner, C. Bellamy, P. L. Amlot, D. Kelly, A. MacGilchrist, M. K. Gandhi, A. J. Swerdlow, and D. H. Crawford. 2007. "Allogeneic cytotoxic T-cell therapy for EBV-positive posttransplantation lymphoproliferative disease: results of a phase 2 multicenter clinical trial." *Blood* 110 (4):1123-31. doi: 10.1182/blood-2006-12-063008.

[59] Prockop, S., E. Doubrovina, S. Suser, G. Heller, J. Barker, P. Dahi, M. A. Perales, E. Papadopoulos, C. Sauter, H. Castro-Malaspina, F. Boulad, K. J. Curran, S. Giralt, B. Gyurkocza, K. C. Hsu, A. Jakubowski, A. M. Hanash, N. A. Kernan, R. Kobos, G. Koehne, H. Landau, D. Ponce, B. Spitzer, J. W. Young, G. Behr, M. Dunphy, S. Haque, J. Teruya-Feldstein, M. Arcila, C. Moung, S. Hsu, A. Hasan, and R. J. O'Reilly. 2020. "Off-the-shelf EBV-specific T cell

immunotherapy for rituximab-refractory EBV-associated lymphoma following transplantation." *J Clin Invest* 130 (2):733-747. doi: 10.1172/JCI121127.

[60] *Rituximab and LMP-Specific T-Cells in Treating Pediatric Solid Organ Recipients with EBV-Positive, CD20-Positive Post-Transplant Lymphoproliferative Disorder*. https://clinicaltrials.gov/ct2/show/nct02900976. Last updated December 23, 2020. Accessed March 2021

[61] Dalton, T., E. Doubrovina, D. Pankov, R. Reynolds, H. Scholze, A. Selvakumar, T. Vizconde, B. Savalia, V. Dyomin, C. Weigel, C. C. Oakes, A. Alonso, O. Elemento, H. Pan, J. M. Phillip, R. J. O'Reilly, B. E. Gewurz, E. Cesarman, and L. Giulino-Roth. 2020. "Epigenetic reprogramming sensitizes immunologically silent EBV+ lymphomas to virus-directed immunotherapy." *Blood* 135 (21):1870-1881. doi: 10.1182/blood.2019004126.

[62] Kazi, S., A. Mathur, G. Wilkie, K. Cheal, R. Battle, N. McGowan, N. Fraser, E. Hargreaves, D. Turner, J. D. M. Campbell, M. Turner, and M. A. Vickers. 2019. "Long-term follow up after third-party viral-specific cytotoxic lymphocytes for immunosuppression- and Epstein-Barr virus-associated lymphoproliferative disease." *Haematologica* 104 (8):e356-e359. doi: 10.3324/haematol.2018.207548.

[63] Schuster, S. J., J. Svoboda, E. A. Chong, S. D. Nasta, A. R. Mato, O. Anak, J. L. Brogdon, I. Pruteanu-Malinici, V. Bhoj, D. Landsburg, M. Wasik, B. L. Levine, S. F. Lacey, J. J. Melenhorst, D. L. Porter, and C. H. June. 2017. "Chimeric Antigen Receptor T Cells in Refractory B-Cell Lymphomas." *N Engl J Med* 377 (26):2545-2554. doi: 10.1056/NEJMoa1708566.

[64] Strati, P., A. Varma, S. Adkins, L. J. Nastoupil, J. Westin, F. B. Hagemeister, N. H. Fowler, H. J. Lee, L. E. Fayad, F. Samaniego, S. Ahmed, Y. Chen, S. Horowitz, S. Arafat, S. Johncy, P. Kebriaei, V. E. Mulanovich, E. Ariza Heredia, and S. S. Neelapu. 2020. "Hematopoietic recovery and immune reconstitution after axicabta-

gene ciloleucel in patients with large B-cell lymphoma." *Haematologica*. doi: 10.3324/haematol.2020.254045.

[65] Locke, F. L., A. Ghobadi, C. A. Jacobson, D. B. Miklos, L. J. Lekakis, O. O. Oluwole, Y. Lin, I. Braunschweig, B. T. Hill, J. M. Timmerman, A. Deol, P. M. Reagan, P. Stiff, I. W. Flinn, U. Farooq, A. Goy, P. A. McSweeney, J. Munoz, T. Siddiqi, J. C. Chavez, A. F. Herrera, N. L. Bartlett, J. S. Wiezorek, L. Navale, A. Xue, Y. Jiang, A. Bot, J. M. Rossi, J. J. Kim, W. Y. Go, and S. S. Neelapu. 2019. "Long-term safety and activity of axicabtagene ciloleucel in refractory large B-cell lymphoma (ZUMA-1): a single-arm, multicentre, phase 1-2 trial." *Lancet Oncol* 20 (1):31-42. doi: 10.1016/S1470-2045(18)30864-7.

[66] Maude, S. L., N. Frey, P. A. Shaw, R. Aplenc, D. M. Barrett, N. J. Bunin, A. Chew, V. E. Gonzalez, Z. Zheng, S. F. Lacey, Y. D. Mahnke, J. J. Melenhorst, S. R. Rheingold, A. Shen, D. T. Teachey, B. L. Levine, C. H. June, D. L. Porter, and S. A. Grupp. 2014. "Chimeric antigen receptor T cells for sustained remissions in leukemia." *N Engl J Med* 371 (16):1507-17. doi: 10.1056/NEJMoa1407222.

[67] Zeng, C., J. Cheng, T. Li, J. Huang, C. Li, L. Jiang, J. Wang, L. Chen, X. Mao, L. Zhu, Y. Lou, J. Zhou, and X. Zhou. 2020. "Efficacy and toxicity for CD22/CD19 chimeric antigen receptor T-cell therapy in patients with relapsed/refractory aggressive B-cell lymphoma involving the gastrointestinal tract." *Cytotherapy* 22 (3):166-171. doi: 10.1016/j.jcyt.2020.01.008.

[68] Avigdor, A., R. Shouval, E. Jacoby, T. Davidson, A. Shimoni, M. Besser, and A. Nagler. 2018. "CAR T cells induce a complete response in refractory Burkitt Lymphoma." *Bone Marrow Transplant* 53 (12):1583-1585. doi: 10.1038/s41409-018-0235-0.

[69] Du, J., and Y. Zhang. 2020. "Sequential anti-CD19, 22, and 20 autologous chimeric antigen receptor T-cell (CAR-T) treatments of a child with relapsed refractory Burkitt lymphoma: a case report and literature review." *J Cancer Res Clin Oncol* 146 (8):2177. doi: 10.1007/s00432-020-03269-9.

[70] Minard, V., L. Shannon, S. Maude, J. Buechner, J. Krueger, F. Locatelli, A. Attarbaschi, T. Laetsch, B. González Martínez, C. Diaz de Heredia Rubio, R. Awasthi, S. Newsome, J. Davis, L. Bubuteishvili-Pacaud, and B. Burkhardt. 2020. "Bianca: Phase II, single-arm, global trial to determine efficacy and safety of tisagenlecleucel in pediatric/young adult (YA) patients (Pts) with relapsed/refractory B-cell non-Hodgkin lymphoma (R/R B-NHL*)."* *Journal of Clinical Oncology* 38 (15_suppl):e22504-e22504. doi: 10.1200/JCO.2020.38.15_suppl.e22504.

[71] Krishnamoorthy, S., A. Ghobadi, R. D. Santos, J. D. Schilling, A. F. Malone, H. Murad, N. L. Bartlett, and T. Alhamad. 2021. "CAR-T therapy in solid organ transplant recipients with treatment refractory posttransplant lymphoproliferative disorder." *Am J Transplant* 21 (2):809-814. doi: 10.1111/ajt.16367.

[72] Wang, T., M. Feng, C. Luo, X. Wan, C. Pan, J. Tang, F. Xue, M. Yin, D. Lu, Q. Xia, B. Li, and J. Chen. 2021. "Successful Treatment of Pediatric Refractory Burkitt Lymphoma PTLD after Liver Transplantation using Anti-CD19 Chimeric Antigen Receptor T-Cell Therapy." *Cell Transplant* 30:963689721996649. doi: 10.1177/0963689721996649.

[73] Worch, J., M. Rohde, and B. Burkhardt. 2013. "Mature B-cell lymphoma and leukemia in children and adolescents-review of standard chemotherapy regimen and perspectives." *Pediatr Hematol Oncol* 30 (6):465-83. doi: 10.3109/08880018.2013.783891.

[74] Minard-Colin, V., L. Brugieres, A. Reiter, M. S. Cairo, T. G. Gross, W. Woessmann, B. Burkhardt, J. T. Sandlund, D. Williams, M. Pillon, K. Horibe, A. Auperin, M. C. Le Deley, M. Zimmerman, S. L. Perkins, M. Raphael, L. Lamant, W. Klapper, L. Mussolin, H. A. Poirel, E. Macintyre, C. Damm-Welk, A. Rosolen, and C. Patte. 2015. "Non-Hodgkin Lymphoma in Children and Adolescents: Progress Through Effective Collaboration, Current Knowledge, and Challenges Ahead." *J Clin Oncol* 33 (27):2963-74. doi: 10.1200/JCO.2014.59.5827.

[75] Windebank, K., T. Walwyn, R. Kirk, G. Parry, A. Hasan, N. Bown, and B. Wilkins. 2009. "Post cardiac transplantation lymphoproliferative disorder presenting as t(8;14) Burkitt leukaemia/lymphoma treated with low intensity chemotherapy and rituximab." *Pediatr Blood Cancer* 53 (3):392-6. doi: 10.1002/pbc.22070.

[76] Xicoy, B., J. M. Ribera, J. Esteve, S. Brunet, M. A. Sanz, P. Fernandez-Abellan, and E. Feliu. 2003. "Post-transplant Burkitt's leukemia or lymphoma. Study of five cases treated with specific intensive therapy (PETHEMA ALL-3/97 trial)." *Leuk Lymphoma* 44 (9):1541-3. doi: 10.3109/10428190309178777.

[77] Zimmermann, H., H. Xu, A. Barlev, A., Feng, W. Navarro, and R. U. Trappe. "Clinical outcomes of solid organ transplant patients with EBV+PTLD who fail first-line rituximab or rituximab plus chemotherapy: an analysis of German PTLD registry." *European Hematology Association* 2019; 266518; PF719.

[78] Anoop, P., S. Sankpal, C. Stiller, S. Tewari, D. L. Lancaster, K. Khabra, and M. M. Taj. 2012. "Outcome of childhood relapsed or refractory mature B-cell non-Hodgkin lymphoma and acute lymphoblastic leukemia." *Leuk Lymphoma* 53 (10):1882-8. doi: 10.3109/10428194.2012.677534.

[79] Woessmann, W., M. Zimmermann, A. Meinhardt, S. Muller, H. Hauch, F. Knorr, I. Oschlies, W. Klapper, F. Niggli, E. Kabickova, A. Attarbaschi, A. Reiter, and B. Burkhardt. 2020. "Progressive or relapsed Burkitt lymphoma or leukemia in children and adolescents after BFM-type first-line therapy." *Blood* 135 (14):1124-1132. doi: 10.1182/blood.2019003591.

[80] Cairo, M., A. Auperin, S. L. Perkins, R. Pinkerton, L. Harrison, S. Goldman, and C. Patte. 2018. "Overall survival of children and adolescents with mature B cell non-Hodgkin lymphoma who had refractory or relapsed disease during or after treatment with FAB/LMB 96: A report from the FAB/LMB 96 study group." *Br J Haematol* 182 (6):859-869. doi: 10.1111/bjh.15491.

[81] AbdelHameid, D., A. Felice, L. B. Cooper, and S. B. Katugaha. 2020. "Long-term remission in an adult heart transplant recipient with advanced Burkitt's lymphoma post-transplant lymphoproliferative disorder after anthracycline-free chemotherapy: A case report and literature review." *Transpl Infect Dis* 22 (4):e13265. doi: 10.1111/tid.13265.

[82] Naik, S., K. Tayapongsak, K. Robbins, C. K. Manavi, M. J. Pettenati, and D. D. Grier. 2013. "Burkitt's Lymphoma Presenting as Late-Onset Posttransplant Lymphoproliferative Disorder following Kidney and Pancreas Transplantation: Case Report and Review of the Literature." *Case Rep Oncol* 6 (1):6-14. doi: 10.1159/000346346.

[83] Paul, J., and B. Francis. 2018. "An unusual presentation of Burkitt lymphoma in a renal allograft recipient." *Journal of Integrative Nephrology and Andrology* 5 (3):116-120. doi: 10.4103/jina.jina_29_17.

[84] Law, M. F., H. N. Chan, C. Leung, H. K. Lai, C. Y. Ha, C. Ng, Y. M. Yeung, and S. F. Yip. 2014. "Burkitt-like post-transplant lymphoproliferative disorder (PTLD) presenting with breast mass in a renal transplant recipient: a report of a rare case." *Ann Hematol* 93 (12):2083-5. doi: 10.1007/s00277-014-2094-0.

[85] Mainardi, V., S. Gerona, G. Ardao, N. Ferreira, G. Ramirez, J. Arbiza, and S. Mirazo. 2019. "Locally Acquired Chronic Hepatitis E Followed by Epstein-Barr Virus Reactivation and Burkitt Lymphoma as a Suspected Extrahepatic Manifestation in a Liver Transplant Recipient." *Am J Case Rep* 20:1016-1021. doi: 10.12659/AJCR.916253.

[86] Akar Ozkan, E., B. H. Ozdemir, A. Akdur, E. E. Deniz, and M. Haberal. 2014. "Burkitt lymphoma after transplant: an aggressive lymphoproliferative disease." *Exp Clin Transplant* 12 Suppl 1:136-8.

In: Burkitt Lymphoma
Editor: Douglas V. Berthelot

ISBN: 978-1-68507-071-7

Chapter 4

BURKITT LYMPHOMA

Luis M. Juárez-Salcedo*[1], *MD,
Diego Conde-Royo*[2], *MD and Samir Dalia*[3], *MD

[1]Department of Hematology,
Gregorio Marañón University Hospital, Madrid, Spain
[2]Department of Hematology,
Principe de Asturias University Hospital, Madrid, Spain
[3]Department of Hematology/Oncology,
Mercy Clinic Oncology and Hematology, Missouri, US

ABSTRACT

Burkitt lymphoma (BL) is an uncommon mature B cell non-Hodgkin lymphoma (NHL) characterized by aggressive clinical behavior with high survival rates among children and young adults. Three different variants are well recognized which differ in epidemiology, clinical presentation, and molecular or biological features. Endemic, sporadic and immunodeficiency-associated are these BL epidemiological forms. The genetic hallmark is the rearrangement of the MYC oncogene, virtually presented in all BL cases. Translocation with the immunoglobulin heavy chain gene region, t(8;14)(q24;q32), is the most frequent (80%). Recently, promising findings by RNA sequencing studies have expanded the molecular landscape with the identification of novel genes probably involved in its pathogenesis. Mutations in the transcription factor TCF3 or ID3 (its negative regulator) have been described in endemic, sporadic, and immunodeficiency-associated BL. Clinical presentation differs according to the epidemiologic variants with nodal and extranodal involvement (central nervous system, bone marrow, gastrointestinal tract). Tumor lysis syndrome, before or after treatment, is frequent because of the massive proliferation rate of BL, being mandatory an appropriate prophylaxis. Initial chemotherapy approaches were based on acute lymphoblastic leukemia intensive pediatrics regimens showing high efficacy in young patients while significant toxicity in older and immunocompromised patients.

Addition of anti CD20 therapy to chemotherapy improved previous outcomes becoming the standard of care in BL. Optimize chemotherapy regimens to decrease toxicity, relapsed/refractory approaches, and incorporate biological findings on treatment are the main goal of the new era of BL management. In this chapter, we will describe the main aspects of this entity, focusing on the pathobiology and the treatment both, in the first-line and relapsed/refractory cases, besides describing the new therapeutic strategies, which in the long term, could improve the results in this pathology.

INTRODUCTION

BL is an aggressive B cell lymphoma which arise from mature germinal or post germinal center B cells. It was originally described in 1958 in Ugandan children, the endemic BL; subsequently, sporadic and immunodeficiency-associated BL were proposed. These three main types harbor the rearrangement of the MYC oncogene, its genetic signature.

Burkitt cell acute lymphoblastic leukemia represents the leukemic form of BL according to the 2016 revised version of the World Health Organization classification (WHO). However, some modifications in the BL category were presented. A subset of BL cases lacking a MYC translocation was defined as a provisional entity called "Burkitt-like Lymphoma with 11q aberration." Likewise, other new subgroup among aggressive B cell lymphomas was proposed, the high-grade B cell lymphomas (HGBLs). Encompassing the latter one, BL cases harboring MYC and BCL2 and/or BCL6 rearrangements or those that do not fulfill the BL category will be included in "HGBLs with MYC and BCL2 and/or

BCL6 rearrangements" and "HGBLs not otherwise specified," respectively (Swerdlow et al. 2016a).

EPIDEMIOLOGY

Three distinct clinical forms of BL are recognized, which overall present different geographical distribution, molecular characteristics and clinical features: endemic, sporadic and immunodeficiency-associated BL. The endemic variant occurs in holoendemic malaria regions of Papua New Guinea and equatorial Africa being associated with Epstein Barr Virus (EBV) infection in virtually all cases.

Endemic BL is the most frequent childhood cancer, encompassing 50% of childhood cancers and 90% of all childhood lymphomas. The median age of diagnosis is 6 years with an incidence peak ranging from 4 to 7 years and a male to female ratio of 2:1 (I. Magrath 2012). An estimated incidence of 3-6 cases per 100.000 children per year has been reported.

Sporadic BL is found generally in Western Europe and United States, accounts 1-2% of adults lymphomas and 30% of pediatric lymphomas (Morton et al. 2006) (Olszewski, Fallah, and Castillo 2016). These areas present an estimated incidence of 2-3 cases per million persons per year (Sant et al. 2010). Association with EBV infection is less common (10-20%) with no specific demographic feature defining this subtype. Median age of adult patients is 30 years whereas among pediatric population there is a peak incidence at the age of 11 years. Male predominance was described with a male and female ratio of 4:1 (Boerma et al. 2004).

Immunodeficiency-associated BL is mainly diagnosed in patients with human immunodeficiency virus (HIV) infection and represents 40% of all lymphomas diagnosed in patients with this condition. Despite the use of active retroviral therapy, the incidence of BL has not decreased unlike other NHLs HIV-related (diffuse large B cell lymphoma [DLBCL] and primary CNS lymphoma) and patients have a 10-20% lifetime risk of developing it (Atallah-Yunes, Murphy, and Noy 2020). Typically, it occurs with a relatively normal CD4 T cell counts (>200 cells/µL), as these cells may be needed for the activation of B-cell germinal centers and subsequent MYC translocation acquisition (Dolcetti et al. 2016). EBV infection was reported in <40% of HIV-associated BL in Europe and United States patients. BL associated to other causes of immunodeficiency is less common with an increased risk after 5 years of organ transplantation. The incidence of immunodeficiency-associated BL in United States is 22 cases per 100,000 patients per year.

PATHOBIOLOGY

BL is derived from germinal or post- germinal center B cells. This is supported by the recognition of a suitable cell immunophenotype with B-cell and germinal center-associated antigens (CD19, CD20, CD79a, CD10 and BCL6) along with the identification of somatic mutations in the variable region of the immunoglobulin genes (IgV) (Swerdlow et al. 2016a).

Furthermore, different findings suggest that BL variants (endemic, sporadic and immunodeficiency-associated) may be originated from B cells at different stages of growth. EBV-negative BL presents low levels of somatic mutation in their IgV heavy chain genes without antigen selection, which correlates with an early centroblast. Meanwhile, EBV-positive BL may be derived from late germinal center B cell or memory B cell as they show higher levels of somatic mutations of IgV heavy chain genes accompanied by antigen selection (Piccaluga et al. 2011).

BL is defined by impaired regulation and translocation of the MYC gene on chromosome 8. The protein encoded by MYC gene is an ongogenic transcription factor involved in several cellular processes like growth, division, proliferation and death, among others. MYC rearrangements are presented in the vast majority of BL. The most common translocation (80%) is t(8;14)(q24;q32), between MYC gene and the immunoglobulin heavy chain gene region on chromosome 14. Less frequent are those concerning the kappa light chain gene (chromosome 2) and lambda light chain gene (chromosome 22), resulting in the t(2;8)(p11;q24) and t(8;22)(q24;q11) found in 15% and 5% of BL respectively (Dalla-Favera et al. 1982) (Swerdlow et al. 2016a). These translocations promote the MYC overexpression, a defining event on BL pathogenesis. However, MYC rearrangements need other partner for BL oncogenesis since up to 5% of BL lack those translocations exhibiting the remaining typical features of BL. Furthermore, other NHLs like DLBCL also carry translocations of the MYC gene. Thus, additional mutations on oncogenes or tumor suppressors together with alternative mechanisms must complement MYC dysregulation. MYC is the gene most frequent mutated in BL, most of them impair MYC removal or MYC dependent-apoptosis through P53 or BIM (pro-apoptotic proteins) (Bahram et al. 2000) (Hemann et al. 2005).

Studies of gene expression and mutational profile of BL described additional molecular abnormalities implicated on BL pathogenesis. Somatic mutations in the ID3 gene (gain of function) or in the TCF3 gene (loss of function) have been reported in 40%, 67% and 70-90% of endemic, immunodeficiency-associated and sporadic BL, respectively (Schmitz et al. 2012) (Love et al. 2012) (Rohde et al. 2017). TCF3 gene is implicated in the modulation of germinal center genes being expressed in the dark zone. TCF3 gene encodes E2A, a transcription factor that promotes cell proliferation and survival via the BCR/PI3K signaling pathway through downregulation of SYK inhibitor SHP-1. This mechanism demonstrates the presence of tonic activity in BL which differs from chronic signaling in the absence of Nf-κB and Bruton's tyrosine kinase activity (Young and Staudt 2013) (Corso et al. 2016). ID3 is the TCF3 inhibitor that allows the transition of the germinal center cells to the light zone. The negative feedback loop of ID3 is compromised by inactivating mutations mostly concentrated in its TCF3 binding region (Panea et al. 2019). Also, TCF3 upregulates CCND3 and up to 30% of BL cases harbor mutations on CCND3 that enhance intracellular cyclin D3 levels leading to cell cycle downregulation (Rohde et al. 2017).

Finally, polymicrobial infections appear to play a role in BL development. Chronic EBV infection occurs essentially in all cases of endemic BL, however its pathologic role is poorly understood. It has been hypothesized that EBV infection may stimulate B cell expansion inhibiting premalignant B cell apoptosis and allowing MYC translocation acquisition (Schmitz et al. 2012). Furthermore, EBV infection displays a latent infection phenotype defined by lack of expression of the transforming proteins LMP-1 and EBNA-2, differing from other EBV related-lymphomas (Vockerodt et al. 2015). Infections like HIV, malaria or arboviruses promote a persistent acute phase of initial EBV infection which allows B cell expansion (Swerdlow et al. 2016a). Recent malaria infection diagnosed by the determination of anti-HRP-II antibodies has been associated with childhood endemic BL with greater probability than long-term malaria infection (Aka et al. 2013). The association between HIV-infection and lymphomagenesis is well described, however its mechanisms are not completely understood. Tat is an HIV protein that has pleiotropic effects in B-cell lymphomagenesis, indeed several studies have described a potential role in BL development. Tat triggers AICDA gene expression which creates double-strand breaks for immunoglobulin gene maturation. It has been reported that Tat increase the proportion of colocalization (spatial overlap between two different fluorescent labels to prove that are located in the same area of the cell) between MYC and IgV heavy chain genes. Finally, DNA damage was reported in both genes (Sall et al. 2019).

A better understanding of BL pathogenesis and the microbial oncogenicity might highlight possible new targets allowing a future therapy landscape.

Clinical Presentation

Clinical presentation may vary according to the BL variant. Nonetheless, BL is characterized by rapid growth with a very short doubling time (24 and 48 hours) and rapid spread to extranodal sites such as the CNS and bone marrow. For this reason, the majority of newly diagnosed patients (> 70%) have advanced Ann Arbor stage III or IV disease. The association of the presentation with the tumor lysis syndrome (TLS) is frequent, which is why a rapid intervention and, in many cases, transfer to the intensive care unit is necessary.

Three distinct clinical forms have been described: endemic, sporadic, and immunodeficiency-associated (Blum, Lozanski, and Byrd 2004).

1. In the endemic (African) form, the greatest involvement is at the mandibular region or facial bone (about 50-60% of cases). Primary involvement of the abdomen, lymph nodes, mediastinum, and spleen are less common. The primary tumor can spread to other extranodal sites, such as the mesentery, ovary, testis, kidney, breast, and meninges. Bone marrow involvement is seen in less than 10% of patients at initial presentation, but it is a common complication of recurrent or refractory disease (I. T. Magrath 1991).
2. The non-endemic (sporadic) form generally has an abdominal presentation (involvement of the distal ileum, stomach, cecum, and/or mesentery), but also affects the kidney, testis, ovary, breast, bone marrow, or central nervous system (CNS) (Ok and Medeiros 2020). Symptoms may include those related to intestinal obstruction or gastrointestinal bleeding, similar to acute appendicitis or intussusception symptoms. Lymphadenopathy, if present, is usually localized. Bone marrow and CNS involvement occur in approximately 30 and 15 percent of initial cases, respectively, at presentation, but they are common complications of relapsed or refractory disease. About 25% of cases will have involvement of the jaw or facial bones (Blum, Lozanski, and Byrd 2004).
3. Patients with BL associated with immunodeficiency primarily present with signs or symptoms related to the underlying immunodeficiency (eg, AIDS, congenital immunodeficiency,

acquired immunodeficiency due to solid or hematopoietic organ transplantation). Cases related to immunodeficiency most often involve the lymph nodes, bone marrow, and CNS.

DIAGNOSIS

The combination of clinical presentation, laboratory tests, imaging studies and results derived from tissue biopsy (histology, immunophenotype and genetic work-up) grant an accurate diagnosis.

Patients should be questioned about systemic symptoms, and their performance status should be assessed. It is important to determine if there is a history of potential causative factors such as prior malignancy, chemotherapy or radiation treatment, or autoimmune or immunodeficiency diseases. A history of infection with or exposure to various pathogens, including HIV and hepatitis B and C, should be excluded. A detailed physical examination should be performed with particular attention to lymph node regions (Swerdlow et al. 2016b).

Laboratory tests should include a complete blood count and serum chemistry. Due to the high proliferation behavior of BL ruling out TLS is crucial. Thus, is necessary to include lactate dehydrogenase (LDH), uric acid and ions (phosphorus, calcium and potassium). As well, HIV and hepatitis serology test in conjunction with Epstein-Barr virus loads may also be useful (Cheson et al. 2014). All patients should undergo lumbar puncture with evaluation of the cerebrospinal fluid by cytology and flow cytometry (Dunleavy and Wilson, n.d.).

An accurate histologic diagnosis is imperative to determine the patient's prognosis and treatment; therefore, the single most important diagnosis test is a properly evaluated and technically adequate excisional tissue biopsy. With few exceptions, fine-needle aspiration is inadequate for diagnosis. Aggressive lymphoma should be diagnosed by an experienced hematopathologist familiar with lymphoma diagnosis in order to improve the results.

Histologic features include cells of intermediate size and basophilic cytoplasm with small vacuoles. A round nuclei and dark nucleoli surrounded by granular chromatin. The distinctive hallmark is a starry-sky pattern, with the basophilic tumor cells as "sky" and macrophages as "stars" (Swerdlow et al. 2016a). The antigen expression in BL cells encompass B-cell and germinal center markers: CD19, CD20, CD22, CD79a, PAX5, CD10 and BCL6. In addition, membrane IgM with light chain restriction together with a Ki-67 proliferation rate nearly 100% are also present (Swerdlow et al. 2016a).

In addition to routine laboratory, imaging studies are important to determine sites of disease involvement (Cheson 2011). Computed tomography (CT) scan of the chest, abdomen and pelvis are necessary. The need for additional imaging studies such as magnetic resonance imaging (MRI) and FDG-PET scanning depends on the clinical presentation and sites of disease (A. Noy et al. 2009). If CNS involvement is highly suspected, evaluation of the head by CT or MRI may be indicated. A BM aspirate should be performed in all patients (Lister et al. 1989).

PROGNOSIS

The Ann Arbor classification is widely used for staging in adults. There is no validated prognostic score in BL but population-based studies have identified prognostic factors such as age, black race, advanced stage, performance stage, and elevated lactate dehydrogenase (LDH) (Castillo and Nadeem 2014)(Tove Wästerlid et al. 2011). Many studies have identified a low-risk category of BL characterized by normal LDH; Eastern Cooperative Oncology Group performance status 0 or 1; Ann Arbor stage 1 or II plus no mass size greater than 7 or 10 cm (Mead et al. 2002).

Treatment

Burkitt lymphoma is a systematic disease and requires chemotherapy for all disease stages. Locoregional radiation does not improve survival and should be avoided.

First-Line Therapy for BL

Since BL has a high rate of replication and growth, it is necessary to use intensive chemotherapy regimens similar to those used in B-ALL that use dose-intense and prolonged treatment with induction, consolidation and maintenance phases (Blum, Lozanski, and Byrd 2004). The regimens used in DLBCL, such as R-CHOP (rituximab, cyclophosphamide, doxorubicin, vincristine, and prednisone), are not recommended due to the low response rates and high probability of relapse (T. Wästerlid et al. 2013).

BL regimens commonly use multiple chemotherapy agents in high doses and alternating cycles. The typically include anthracyclines, epipodophyllotoxinsm, vinca alkaloids, and alkylators, as well as methotrexate and cytarabine, which are cell cycle active agents and take advantage of the high tumor proliferation. These agents, however, are administered in a variety of combinations and schedule, indicating the empiric nature of the actual combinations.

However, there remains a therapeutic challenge in older and immunocompromised patients with BL due to poor tolerability of intensive approaches. The search for risk adapted therapy (where lower-risk patients receive less-intensive regimens) has been helpful in some studies but there remains an unmet need to develop optimal approaches that maintain high cure rates with low toxicity in these populations. The inclusion of Rituximab into the first-line chemotherapy has improved the results obtained by QT and many low dose regimens have exchanged the dose intensity for pharmacokinetically (Hoelzer et al. 2014).

There are multiple highly effective regimens for BL, as R-hyper CVAD (rituximab, cyclophosphamide, vincristine, doxorubicin, and dexamethasone alternating with high-dose methotrexate and cytarabine). The addition of rituximab to the classical B-ALL regimen increased the CR to 86% of cases and 3-years OS to 89% (Thomas et al. 2006), and has also been applied in the HIV BL. However, it has proven difficult to deliver outside of centers of expertise, requiring over 6 months of high-intensity chemotherapy with severe myelosuppression and TRM in 12% of patients (Short et al. 2017).

The CODOX-M/IVAC regimen (cyclophosphamide, doxorubicin, vincristine/ ifosfamide, cytarabine, and etoposide), also called Magrath regimen, was initially developed at the National Cancer Institute in the 1980s for the treatment of aggressive NHL. In 2002, Mead et al. reported the results of 2 alternating cycles of CODOX-M and IVAC for high-risk BL, and 3 cycles of CODOX-M in low risk patients. In high-risk BL, 2-year OS of 70% and EFS of 60% were achieved, but with high rates of severe mucositis and myelosuppression (Mead et al. 2002). Likewise, Lacasce et al, in a phase 2 study described a 'modified Magrath' regimen using altered doses and timing of agents, with 90% CR and 64% disease-free survival (DFS) at 29 months, with no grade 3/4 neuropathy and only one patient had grade 3/4 mucositis. Rituximab was added to this regimen in a retrospective study, demonstrating fewer relapses (7% vs. 33%), better 3-year PFS (74% vs. 61%), and OS (77% vs. 66%) (Lacasce et al. 2004).

Toxicity is an important clinical limitation of these regimens in adults, particularly in the elderly and immunosuppressed patients, due to the associated toxicity and high mortality rates. Therefore, one of the main therapeutic challenges in BL is to develop therapies that are as effective in achieving high cure rates as "standard" regimens, but also improve the therapeutic index and reduce toxicity complications. This approach has been investigated in a study using DA-EPOCH-R regimen. Dunleavy et al. in 2006 reported the outcome of 19 patients with HIV-negative BL treated with this regimen besides CNS prophylaxis with 8 doses of intrathecal methotrexate. After a median follow-up of 86 months, the rate of progression-free survival was 95% (95% CI 75 to 99%) and an OS rate of

100% (95% CI 82 to 100%). Similar regimens like the SC-EPOCH-RR version were probed in patients with BL, at median follow- up of >5 years, rates of freedom from progression (FFP) and OS were 100% and 90%, respectively (Dunleavy et al. 2013).

Nowadays, both, DA-R-EPOCH or HyperCVAD regimens are the most recommended chemotherapy combinations for the first line treatment of BL, due the good results obtained and low complications rates.

Treatment Regimen in the Context of CNS Involvement

To date, there are no data on the high intensity chemotherapy regimen that presents better results in the management of BL with CNS involvement. The lower intensity DAEPOCH-R regimen is an important conceptual advance, particularly for older or HIV-positive patients, who historically had poor tolerance and worse outcomes with dose-intensive chemotherapy. A recent retrospective of 557 adult patients with BL treated in the US suggested that there were no differences in PFS or OS between patients receiving hyperCVAD, CODOX-M / IVAC, or DA-EPOCH explaining baseline prognostic factors (age, LDH, functional status and CNS involvement). Rates of CNS involvement in the BL are 14% to 41% at presentation and 6% to 42% at relapse. BL, similar to B-ALL, is prone to leptomeningeal spread and, based on historical data, most cases of CNS involvement were leptomeningeal, warranting a focus on IT therapy (Sariban et al. 1983).

Although intensive CNS therapy can eradicate BL from the CNS compartment, the median survival after relapse is <3 months. Consequently, all BL regimens include CNS-specific prophylaxis, DA-EPOCH-R has the same or greater intensity of IT injections than hyperCVAD and CODOX-M/IVAC, but lacks the classical agents (methotrexate, cytarabine) used for prophylaxis against parenchymal CNS disease. Similar conclusions emerged from the multi-institutional retrospective, where recurrences in the CNS were more frequent after DA-EPOCH (12%) than with hyperCVAD or CODOX-M/IVAC (3-4%). Risk factors for CNS recurrence included baseline CNS involvement and stage 4 disease. As a result, the adoption of DA-EPOCH-R as first-line treatment has been limited and many centers favor high-intensity regimens for patients with CNS risk factors. We favor R-CODOX-M/IVAC due to its shorter duration and early IT therapy when DA-EPOCH-R is used (Zayac and Olszewski 2020).

Treatment of Relapsed and Refractory BL

Although standard first-line chemotherapy regimens show high rates of CR and PFS, there are 20% to 40% of patients who are refractory or relapsing. In this context, there is insufficient evidence to determine the best treatment strategy.

In patients whose relapse is after 6 months from the initiation therapy, they can achieve a second remission with additional combinations such as ICE (ifosfamide, carboplatin and etoposide), DAEPOCH-R, IVAC, GDP (gemcitabine, dexamethasone and cisplatin) or cytarabine in high doses. They are often given with rituximab and consolidation of results with an autologous or allogeneic stem cell transplant (SCT) is recommended (Sweetenham et al. 1996).

While SCT in the second CR resulted in OS of up to 70% in the pre-rituximab era, most BL patients experience an early chemotherapy-resistant relapse and <10% survive a relapse after a high intensity induction. Recent data indicate that patients in the second CR achieve 44% long-term PFS after autologous and 27% after allogeneic SCT, while with a partial response, the 5-year PFS is only 19% and 11%, respectively. ('Transplant Activity Report' 2019).

Given that even with these strategies the results in patients with LB R / R are not encouraging, new therapeutic alternatives with novel approaches are being investigated, but the specific data of BL remains extremely limited. The most promising strategies include immunotherapy (including new cell therapies) or rationally selected targeted therapies.

Targeted Therapies

Based on the molecular pathobiologyy of BL, targeted therapeutic approaches may include inhibition of the B-cell receptor (BCR), PI3K or SYK (directly or indirectly through the chaperone heat-shock protein 90 [HSP90]), disruption of MYC function using inhibitors of proteins with bromodomain and extra-terminal motifs (BET/BRD), deregulation of metabolism (devimistat), or disturbing the proliferation/apoptosis balance by inhibiting cyclin-dependent kinases CDK4/6 or apoptosis regulators like MCL-1. Unfortunately, despite encouraging pre-clinical data, these approaches are only starting to be clinically explored. Abemaciclib and palbociclib, two structurally different CDK4/6 inhibitors, suppress proliferation and induce apoptosis in aggressive NHL cell lines, although the effects of abemaciclib appeared to be greater and more dependent on cyclin D3 expression (Tanaka et al. 2020). JQ1, a small molecule BRD inhibitor, exerted in vitro activity against BL cell lines, and addition of a PI3K/mTOR inhibitor omipalisib augmented this response. Other preclinical observations suggest activity of PI3K/mTOR inhibitors omipalisib and idelalisib, alone or in combination with chemotherapy. Molibresib, a selective BRD/BET inhibitor, showed modest clinical activity in a phase 1 study in relapsed/refractory NHL, but actually not among subjects with BL (Piha-Paul et al. 2019). The MCL-1 inhibitor, AMG-176, showed so far pre-clinical activity against BL cell lines. One novel targeted approach already translated into a clinical study involves disrupting the MYC-driven glycolytic metabolism that relies on the tricarboxylic acid cycle using the novel lipoic acid analog devimistat (CPI-613). Devimistat is being investigated in a phase 2 study following a sustained response observed in a patient with BL (Ariela Noy et al. n.d.).

Chimeric Antigen Receptor (CAR) T-Cell Therapy

A new tool used in the management of lymphoproliferative syndromes is CAR-T therapy, with response rates of 50-90% and long-lasting remissions in 30-40% of patients with relapsed/refractory precursor ALL-B or DLBCL (Neelapu et al. 2017). However, its usefulness in the treatment of BL is not proven since this entity was excluded from most of the CAR-T trials. In that sense, its usefulness remains experimental and without real world data on commercial products (axicabtagene ciloleucel and tisagenlecleucel). The rapid rate of progression of BL would compromise the applicability of CAR T cells. However, new trials on the usefulness of this tool in BL are underway. One of them evaluated the sequential use of CART-cell anti CD-19, CD20 and CD 22 in refractory/relapsed lymphoma, especially in BL, preliminary reporting response rates of 42% after the first infusion and CRs rates of the 71%. Additional targets for CAR T-cells therapy are under investigation, including a molecular anti CD10 CAR T-cell system, and a multiantigen-targeting CAR NK-cell product. And ongoing trial, the CARPALL study of a novel "fast off-rate" anti-CD19 CAR T-cell therapy is recruiting pediatric patients with BL (NCT02443831).

Bispecific T-Cell Engagers (BiTEs)

A BiTE is a recombinant bispecific protein that has two linked scFvs from two different antibodies, one targeting a cell-surface molecule on T cells (for example, CD3 or CD19/CD20) and the other targeting antigens on the surface of malignant cells. Blinatumomab, a CD19/CD3 construct, used in relapses-refractory B-ALL, was used in monotherapy in BL with disappoint results (Kantarjian et al. 2016). An ongoing phase I study is evaluating the combination of Blinatumumab with Lenalidomide in relapsed/refractory NHL, including BL (Poh et al. 2019). Other BiTEs like mosunetuzumab are being studied in different clinical trials (REGN1979 or GEN3013), with promising responses in R/R aggressive NHL (Schuster et al. 2019).

Conclusion

The BL is an uncommon highly aggressive B cell neoplasm characterized by the translocation and deregulation of the MYC gene on chromosome 8. Three distinct clinical forms of BL are recognized: endemic, sporadic, and immunodeficiency-associated. It is a lymphoma with aggressive behavior and growth in a few hours, with a high risk of complications (such as TLS) and with a high mortality rate. A correct pathological diagnosis and molecular alterations are necessary. Currently, intensive immunochemotherapy remains the best therapeutic option. The different treatment regimens used have achieved similar remission rates, but with very high toxicity rates that limit their use. These days, the most recommended regimens are DA-R-EPOCH or HyperCVAD. There are few treatment alternatives in refractory or relapsed cases, consolidation with autologous transplantation, or in specific cases, allogeneic transplantation is indicated. New therapeutic alternatives (targeted therapies) are being explored, still with inconclusive results.

References

Aka, Peter, Maria Candida Vila, Amar Jariwala, Francis Nkrumah, Benjamin Emmanuel, Masanori Yagi, Nirianne Marie Q. Palacpac, et al. 2013. 'Endemic Burkitt Lymphoma Is Associated with Strength and Diversity of Plasmodium Falciparum Malaria Stage-Specific Antigen Antibody Response.' *Blood* 122 (5): 629–35. https://doi.org/10.1182/blood-2012-12-475665.

Atallah-Yunes, Suheil Albert, Dermot J. Murphy, and Ariela Noy. 2020. 'HIV-Associated Burkitt Lymphoma.' *The Lancet. Haematology* 7 (8): e594–600. https://doi.org/10.1016/S2352-3026(20)30126-5.

Bahram, F., N. von der Lehr, C. Cetinkaya, and L. G. Larsson. 2000. 'C-Myc Hot Spot Mutations in Lymphomas Result in Inefficient

Ubiquitination and Decreased Proteasome-Mediated Turnover.' *Blood* 95 (6): 2104–10.

Blum, Kristie A., Gerard Lozanski, and John C. Byrd. 2004. 'Adult Burkitt Leukemia and Lymphoma.' *Blood* 104 (10): 3009–20. https://doi.org/10.1182/blood-2004-02-0405.

Boerma, E. G., G. W. van Imhoff, I. M. Appel, N. J. G. M. Veeger, Ph M. Kluin, and J. C. Kluin-Nelemans. 2004. 'Gender and Age-Related Differences in Burkitt Lymphoma--Epidemiological and Clinical Data from the Netherlands.' *European Journal of Cancer (Oxford, England: 1990)* 40 (18): 2781–87. https://doi.org/10.1016/j.ejca. 2004.09.004.

Castillo, Jorge J, and Omar Nadeem. 2014. 'Improving the Accuracy in Prognosis for Burkitt Lymphoma Patients.' *Expert Review of Anticancer Therapy* 14 (2): 125–27. https://doi.org/10.1586/14737140. 2014.866042.

Cheson, Bruce D. 2011. 'Role of Functional Imaging in the Management of Lymphoma.' *Journal of Clinical Oncology: Official Journal of the American Society of Clinical Oncology* 29 (14): 1844–54. https://doi.org/10.1200/JCO.2010.32.5225.

Cheson, Bruce D., Richard I. Fisher, Sally F. Barrington, Franco Cavalli, Lawrence H. Schwartz, Emanuele Zucca, T. Andrew Lister, et al. 2014. 'Recommendations for Initial Evaluation, Staging, and Response Assessment of Hodgkin and Non-Hodgkin Lymphoma: The Lugano Classification.' *Journal of Clinical Oncology: Official Journal of the American Society of Clinical Oncology* 32 (27): 3059–68. https://doi.org/10.1200/JCO.2013.54.8800.

Corso, Jasmin, Kuan-Ting Pan, Roland Walter, Carmen Doebele, Sebastian Mohr, Hanibal Bohnenberger, Philipp Ströbel, et al. 2016. 'Elucidation of Tonic and Activated B-Cell Receptor Signaling in Burkitt's Lymphoma Provides Insights into Regulation of Cell Survival.' *Proceedings of the National Academy of Sciences of the United States of America* 113 (20): 5688–93. https://doi.org/10.1073/pnas.1601053113.

Dalla-Favera, R., M. Bregni, J. Erikson, D. Patterson, R. C. Gallo, and C. M. Croce. 1982. 'Human C-Myc Onc Gene Is Located on the Region of Chromosome 8 That Is Translocated in Burkitt Lymphoma Cells.' *Proceedings of the National Academy of Sciences of the United States of America* 79 (24): 7824–27. https://doi.org/10.1073/pnas.79.24.7824.

Dolcetti, Riccardo, Annunziata Gloghini, Arnaldo Caruso, and Antonino Carbone. 2016. 'A Lymphomagenic Role for HIV beyond Immune Suppression?' *Blood* 127 (11): 1403–9. https://doi.org/10.1182/blood-2015-11-681411.

Dunleavy, Kieron, Stefania Pittaluga, Lauren S. Maeda, Ranjana Advani, Clara C. Chen, Julie Hessler, Seth M. Steinberg, et al. 2013. 'Dose-Adjusted EPOCH-Rituximab Therapy in Primary Mediastinal B-Cell Lymphoma.' *The New England Journal of Medicine* 368 (15): 1408–16. https://doi.org/10.1056/NEJMoa1214561.

Dunleavy, Kieron, and Wyndham Wilson. n.d. 'Diagnosis and Treatment of Diffuse Large B-Cell Lymphoma and Burkitt Lymphoma.' In *Hematology: Basic Principles and Practice*, 6th ed., 1236–44. Elsevier.

Hemann, Michael T., Anka Bric, Julie Teruya-Feldstein, Andreas Herbst, Jonas A. Nilsson, Carlos Cordon-Cardo, John L. Cleveland, William P. Tansey, and Scott W. Lowe. 2005. 'Evasion of the P53 Tumour Surveillance Network by Tumour-Derived MYC Mutants.' *Nature* 436 (7052): 807–11. https://doi.org/10.1038/nature03845.

Hoelzer, Dieter, Jan Walewski, Hartmut Döhner, Andreas Viardot, Wolfgang Hiddemann, Karsten Spiekermann, Hubert Serve, et al. 2014. 'Improved Outcome of Adult Burkitt Lymphoma/Leukemia with Rituximab and Chemotherapy: Report of a Large Prospective Multicenter Trial.' *Blood* 124 (26): 3870–79. https://doi.org/10.1182/blood-2014-03-563627.

Kantarjian, Hagop M., Anthony S. Stein, Ralf C. Bargou, Carlos Grande Garcia, Richard A. Larson, Matthias Stelljes, Nicola Gökbuget, et al. 2016. 'Blinatumomab Treatment of Older Adults with Relapsed/Refractory B-Precursor Acute Lymphoblastic Leukemia: Results from 2 Phase 2 Studies.' *Cancer* 122 (14): 2178–85. https://doi.org/10.1002/cncr.30031.

Lacasce, A., O. Howard, S. Lib, D. Fisher, A. Weng, D. Neuberg, and M. Shipp. 2004. 'Modified Magrath Regimens for Adults with Burkitt and Burkitt-like Lymphomas: Preserved Efficacy with Decreased Toxicity.' *Leukemia & Lymphoma* 45 (4): 761–67. https://doi.org/10.1080/1042819031000141301.

Lister, T. A., D. Crowther, S. B. Sutcliffe, E. Glatstein, G. P. Canellos, R. C. Young, S. A. Rosenberg, C. A. Coltman, and M. Tubiana. 1989. 'Report of a Committee Convened to Discuss the Evaluation and Staging of Patients with Hodgkin's Disease: Cotswolds Meeting.' *Journal of Clinical Oncology: Official Journal of the American Society of Clinical Oncology* 7 (11): 1630–36. https://doi.org/10.1200/JCO.1989.7.11.1630.

Love, Cassandra, Zhen Sun, Dereje Jima, Guojie Li, Jenny Zhang, Rodney Miles, Kristy L. Richards, et al. 2012. 'The Genetic Landscape of Mutations in Burkitt Lymphoma.' *Nature Genetics* 44 (12): 1321–25. https://doi.org/10.1038/ng.2468.

Magrath, I. T. 1991. 'African Burkitt's Lymphoma. History, Biology, Clinical Features, and Treatment.' *The American Journal of Pediatric Hematology/Oncology* 13 (2): 222–46.

Magrath, Ian. 2012. 'Epidemiology: Clues to the Pathogenesis of Burkitt Lymphoma.' *British Journal of Haematology* 156 (6): 744–56. https://doi.org/10.1111/j.1365-2141.2011.09013.x.

Mead, G. M., M. R. Sydes, J. Walewski, A. Grigg, C. S. Hatton, N. Pescosta, C. Guarnaccia, et al. 2002. 'An International Evaluation of CODOX-M and CODOX-M Alternating with IVAC in Adult Burkitt's Lymphoma: Results of United Kingdom Lymphoma Group LY06 Study.' *Annals of Oncology: Official Journal of the European Society for Medical Oncology* 13 (8): 1264–74. https://doi.org/10.1093/annonc/mdf253.

Morton, Lindsay M., Sophia S. Wang, Susan S. Devesa, Patricia Hartge, Dennis D. Weisenburger, and Martha S. Linet. 2006. 'Lymphoma Incidence Patterns by WHO Subtype in the United States, 1992-2001.' *Blood* 107 (1): 265–76. https://doi.org/10.1182/blood-2005-06-2508.

Neelapu, Sattva S., Frederick L. Locke, Nancy L. Bartlett, Lazaros J. Lekakis, David B. Miklos, Caron A. Jacobson, Ira Braunschweig, et al. 2017. 'Axicabtagene Ciloleucel CAR T-Cell Therapy in Refractory Large B-Cell Lymphoma.' *The New England Journal of Medicine* 377 (26): 2531–44. https://doi.org/10.1056/NEJMoa1707447.

Noy, A., H. Schöder, M. Gönen, M. Weissler, K. Ertelt, C. Cohler, C. Portlock, P. Hamlin, and H. W. D. Yeung. 2009. 'The Majority of Transformed Lymphomas Have High Standardized Uptake Values (SUVs) on Positron Emission Tomography (PET) Scanning Similar to Diffuse Large B-Cell Lymphoma (DLBCL).' *Annals of Oncology* 20 (3): 508–12. https://doi.org/10.1093/annonc/mdn657.

Noy, Ariela, Timothy S Pardee, Liana Nikolenko, Raphael E Steiner, Jeremy Abramson, Kieron Dunleavy, and Sanjeev Luther. n.d. '*A Phase II Clinical Trial of CPI-613® (Devimistat) in Patients with Relapsed or Refractory Burkitt Lymphoma/Leukemia or High-Grade B-Cell Lymphoma with Rearrangements of MYC and BCL2 and/or BCL6 (DHL/THL)*,' 1.

Ok, Chi Young, and L. Jeffrey Medeiros. 2020. 'High-Grade B-Cell Lymphoma: A Term Re-Purposed in the Revised WHO Classification.' *Pathology* 52 (1): 68–77. https://doi.org/10.1016/j.pathol.2019.09.008.

Olszewski, Adam J., Jaleh Fallah, and Jorge J. Castillo. 2016. 'Human Immunodeficiency Virus-Associated Lymphomas in the Antiretroviral Therapy Era: Analysis of the National Cancer Data Base.' *Cancer* 122 (17): 2689–97. https://doi.org/10.1002/cncr.30112.

Panea, Razvan I., Cassandra L. Love, Jennifer R. Shingleton, Anupama Reddy, Jeffrey A. Bailey, Ann M. Moormann, Juliana A. Otieno, et al. 2019. 'The Whole-Genome Landscape of Burkitt Lymphoma Subtypes.' *Blood* 134 (19): 1598–1607. https://doi.org/10.1182/blood.2019001880.

Piccaluga, Pier Paolo, Giulia De Falco, Manjunath Kustagi, Anna Gazzola, Claudio Agostinelli, Claudio Tripodo, Eleonora Leucci, et al. 2011. 'Gene Expression Analysis Uncovers Similarity and Differences among Burkitt Lymphoma Subtypes.' *Blood* 117 (13): 3596–3608. https://doi.org/10.1182/blood-2010-08-301556.

Piha-Paul, Sarina A, Christine L Hann, Christopher A French, Sophie Cousin, Irene Braña, Phillippe A Cassier, Victor Moreno, et al. 2019. 'Phase 1 Study of Molibresib (GSK525762), a Bromodomain and Extra-Terminal Domain Protein Inhibitor, in NUT Carcinoma and Other Solid Tumors.' *JNCI Cancer Spectrum* 4 (2). https://doi.org/10.1093/jncics/pkz093.

Poh, C., P. Frankel, C. Ruel, M. Abedi, E. Schwab, C. Costello, J. Zain, et al. 2019. '*Blinatumomab/Lenalidomide in Relapsed/Refractory Non-Hodgkin's Lymphoma: A Phase I California Cancer Consortium Study of Safety, Efficacy and Immune Correlative Analysis.*' https://doi.org/10.1182/BLOOD-2019-124254.

Rohde, Marius, Bettina R. Bonn, Martin Zimmermann, Jonas Lange, Anja Möricke, Wolfram Klapper, Ilske Oschlies, et al. 2017. 'Relevance of ID3-TCF3-CCND3 Pathway Mutations in Pediatric Aggressive B-Cell Lymphoma Treated According to the Non-Hodgkin Lymphoma Berlin-Frankfurt-Münster Protocols.' *Haematologica* 102 (6): 1091–98. https://doi.org/10.3324/haematol.2016.156885.

Sall, Fatimata Bintou, Rawan El Amine, Diana Markozashvili, Tatyana Tsfasman, Eric Oksenhendler, Marc Lipinski, Yegor Vassetzky, and Diego Germini. 2019. 'HIV-1 Tat Protein Induces Aberrant Activation of AICDA in Human B-Lymphocytes from Peripheral Blood.' *Journal of Cellular Physiology*, January. https://doi.org/10.1002/jcp.28219.

Sant, Milena, Claudia Allemani, Carmen Tereanu, Roberta De Angelis, Riccardo Capocaccia, Otto Visser, Rafael Marcos-Gragera, et al. 2010. 'Incidence of Hematologic Malignancies in Europe by Morphologic Subtype: Results of the HAEMACARE Project.' *Blood* 116 (19): 3724–34. https://doi.org/10.1182/blood-2010-05-282632.

Sariban, E., B. Edwards, C. Janus, and I. Magrath. 1983. 'Central Nervous System Involvement in American Burkitt's Lymphoma.' *Journal of Clinical Oncology: Official Journal of the American Society of Clinical Oncology* 1 (11): 677–81. https://doi.org/10.1200/JCO.1983.1.11.677.

Schmitz, Roland, Ryan M. Young, Michele Ceribelli, Sameer Jhavar, Wenming Xiao, Meili Zhang, George Wright, et al. 2012. 'Burkitt Lymphoma Pathogenesis and Therapeutic Targets from Structural and Functional Genomics.' *Nature* 490 (7418): 116–20. https://doi.org/10.1038/nature11378.

Schuster, Stephen J., Nancy L. Bartlett, Sarit Assouline, Sung Soo Yoon, Francesc Bosch, Laurie H. Sehn, Chan Y. Cheah, et al. 2019. 'Mosunetuzumab Induces Complete Remissions in Poor Prognosis Non-Hodgkin Lymphoma Patients, Including Those Who Are Resistant to or Relapsing After Chimeric Antigen Receptor T-Cell (CAR-T) Therapies, and Is Active in Treatment through Multiple Lines.' *Blood* 134 (1). https://doi.org/10.1182/blood-2019-123742.

Short, Nicholas J., Hagop M. Kantarjian, Heidi Ko, Joseph D. Khoury, Farhad Ravandi, Deborah A. Thomas, Guillermo Garcia-Manero, et al. 2017. 'Outcomes of Adults with Relapsed or Refractory Burkitt and High-Grade B-Cell Leukemia/Lymphoma.' *American Journal of Hematology* 92 (6): E114–17. https://doi.org/10.1002/ajh.24720.

Sweetenham, J. W., R. Pearce, G. Taghipour, D. Blaise, C. Gisselbrecht, and A. H. Goldstone. 1996. 'Adult Burkitt's and Burkitt-like Non-Hodgkin's Lymphoma--Outcome for Patients Treated with High-Dose Therapy and Autologous Stem-Cell Transplantation in First Remission or at Relapse: Results from the European Group for Blood and Marrow Transplantation.' *Journal of Clinical Oncology: Official Journal of the American Society of Clinical Oncology* 14 (9): 2465–72. https://doi.org/10.1200/JCO.1996.14.9.2465.

Swerdlow, Steven H., Elias Campo, Stefano A. Pileri, Nancy Lee Harris, Harald Stein, Reiner Siebert, Ranjana Advani, et al. 2016a. 'The 2016 Revision of the World Health Organization Classification of Lymphoid Neoplasms.' *Blood* 127 (20): 2375–90. https://doi.org/10.1182/blood-2016-01-643569.

———. 2016b. 'The 2016 Revision of the World Health Organization Classification of Lymphoid Neoplasms.' *Blood* 127 (20): 2375–90. https://doi.org/10.1182/blood-2016-01-643569.

Tanaka, Yuka, Shuji Momose, Takayuki Tabayashi, Keisuke Sawada, Takahisa Yamashita, Morihiro Higashi, Morihiko Sagawa, et al. 2020. 'Abemaciclib, a CDK4/6 Inhibitor, Exerts Preclinical Activity against Aggressive Germinal Center-Derived B-Cell Lymphomas.' *Cancer Science* 111 (2): 749–59. https://doi.org/10.1111/cas.14286.

Thomas, Deborah A., Stefan Faderl, Susan O'Brien, Carlos Bueso-Ramos, Jorge Cortes, Guillermo Garcia-Manero, Francis J. Giles, et al. 2006. 'Chemoimmunotherapy with Hyper-CVAD plus Rituximab for the Treatment of Adult Burkitt and Burkitt-Type Lymphoma or Acute Lymphoblastic Leukemia.' *Cancer* 106 (7): 1569–80. https://doi.org/10.1002/cncr.21776.

'Transplant Activity Report.' 2019. *Blood Stem Cell*. 29 October 2019. https://bloodstemcell.hrsa.gov/data/donation-and-transplantation-statistics/transplant-activity-report.

Vockerodt, Martina, Lee-Fah Yap, Claire Shannon-Lowe, Helen Curley, Wenbin Wei, Katerina Vrzalikova, and Paul G. Murray. 2015. 'The Epstein-Barr Virus and the Pathogenesis of Lymphoma.' *The Journal of Pathology* 235 (2): 312–22. https://doi.org/10.1002/path.4459.

Wästerlid, T., P. N. Brown, O. Hagberg, H. Hagberg, L. M. Pedersen, F. D'Amore, and M. Jerkeman. 2013. 'Impact of Chemotherapy Regimen and Rituximab in Adult Burkitt Lymphoma: A Retrospective Population-Based Study from the Nordic Lymphoma Group.' *Annals of Oncology* 24 (7): 1879–86. https://doi.org/10.1093/annonc/mdt058.

Wästerlid, Tove, Björn Jonsson, Hans Hagberg, and Mats Jerkeman. 2011. 'Population Based Study of Prognostic Factors and Treatment in Adult Burkitt Lymphoma: A Swedish Lymphoma Registry Study.' *Leukemia & Lymphoma* 52 (11): 2090–96. https://doi.org/10.3109/10428194.2011.593274.

Young, Ryan M., and Louis M. Staudt. 2013. 'Targeting Pathological B Cell Receptor Signalling in Lymphoid Malignancies.' *Nature Reviews. Drug Discovery* 12 (3): 229–43. https://doi.org/10.1038/nrd3937.

Zayac, Adam S., and Adam J. Olszewski. 2020. 'Burkitt Lymphoma: Bridging the Gap between Advances in Molecular Biology and Therapy.' *Leukemia & Lymphoma* 61 (8): 1784–96. https://doi.org/10.1080/10428194.2020.1747068.

In: Burkitt Lymphoma
Editor: Douglas V. Berthelot
ISBN: 978-1-68507-071-7

Chapter 5

EXAMINING THE THERAPEUTIC ADVANCES FOR BURKITT LYMPHOMA

Daniella E.C.C.O.H Kingsley-Godwin*, MD, PhD,
Maria Jana Kingsley Godwin
and Joshua Kingsley-Godwin, PhD
London Medical Academy, London, England, United Kingdom

ABSTRACT

Burkitt lymphomas are aggressive B-cell cancers (non-Hodgkin type of lymphomas) that frequently involve aggressive progression in the bone marrow and in the central nervous system. Burkitt lymphoma (also known as small non-cleaved cell lymphoma and Burkitt's lymphoma) has a variant termed Burkitt-like lymphoma or BLL. Other types or Burkitt lymphomas are termed: Endemic or African is a type that usually involves the jaw and the facial bones; Sporadic Burkitt lymphoma involves abdominal tumors and Immunodeficiency-related Burkitt lymphoma has lymph node and bone marrow involvement. The World Health Organization suggests that there is little difference between Burkitt lymphoma and BLL and considers them essentially the same

* Corresponding Author's E-mail: daniellagodwin@ymail.com and dkingsley@iahcp.uk.

disease. The order variants are classified under the term Burkitt lymphoma. Due to their rapid progression, these lymphomas are considered medical emergencies that require fast diagnosis and efficient treatment. Hence this clinical systematic review and experts' opinions analyses examines the therapeutic advances in Burkitt lymphoma.

Keywords: Burkitt lymphoma, MYC, Epstein-Barr virus, Rituximab, Burkitt-like lymphoma, therapeutic, treatment, advances

INTRODUCTION

Burkitt lymphoma (BL) is a form of non-Hodgkin's lymphoma (NHL) is cancer, which starts in immune cells called B-cells [1]. BL is recognized as a fast growing human tumor that is associated with impaired immunity and it is rapidly fatal if left untreated [1, 2]. However, intensive chemotherapy can achieve long-tern survival in more than half of the people with BL.

BL is named after British surgeon Denis Burkitt, who first identified this unusual disease in 1956 among children in Africa. In Africa, BL is common in young children who also have malaria and Epstein-Barr virus (EBV) that causes infectious mononucleosis [2]. One mechanism may be that malaria weakens the immune system's response to EBV, allowing it to change infected B-cells into cancerous cells. About 98% of African cases are associated with EBV infection [1-4].

Outside of Africa, BL is rare. In the United States of America (USA), about 1,200 people are diagnosed each year, and about 59% of patients are over age 40 [4, 5]. BL is especially likely to develop in people infected with human immunodeficiency virus (HIV), the virus that causes acquired immune deficiency syndrome (AIDS) [6]. Before highly active antiretroviral therapy (HAART) became a widespread treatment for HIV/AIDS, the incidence of BL was estimated to be 1,000 times higher in HIV-positive people than in the general population [4-6].

In the past years, researchers and scientists have discovered different combinations of treatment regimens, including chemotherapy, and combined them with rituximab as a new form of BL treatment [7-9]. However, resistance can occur in some cases, and there is need for advances in techniques in the diagnosis of BL, and especially in looking into more efficient and effective treatments for it in the changing world. As a result, the purpose of our study is to examine the therapeutic advances for BL using clinical systematic review and experts' opinions analysis method.

METHODS

Clinical systematic review and experts' opinions analysis methods were used in carrying out this study. A literature search of therapeutic advances for BL was performed for peer reviewed articles written in English language, using the electronic databases such as of PubMed, EMBASE, SCOPUS from 1966 to May 2021. In addition, experts' opinions reports and relevant information resources on BL were also obtained and examined. The following search terms were input for the electronic databases search:

1. Burkitt lymphoma or Burkitt's lymphoma (Title/Abstract/full text)
2. Therapy/treatment in (Title/Abstract/full text).
3. Advances in therapy and treatment/managed of Burkitt lymphoma

Experts' opinions reports were also obtained from libraries and health services centers, including at some internet sites.

All authors investigated all relevant studies and reports for quality and publication date. In particular, a list of references was added manually in order to have adequate and relevant information for the study.

RESULTS

The searches yielded 2,215 published materials. After further review and refinements of the articles, reports and information resources, 69 references were selected to be used in conducting this study. The results of the findings from the terms stated in the "methods" section above were group under the following items:

(i) Description of BL
(ii) Etiology/causes of BL
(iii) Types of BL
(iv) Epidemiology of BL
(v) Clinical presentations of BL
(vi) Clinical evaluation of BL
(vii) EBV and BL
(viii) Diagnosis of BL
(ix) Determination of the staging of BL
(x) Histology/Morphology and cytogenetics
(xi) Immunophenotype and molecular signature
(xii) Treatment choices of BL
(xiii) Future directions in MYC inhibition
(xiv) New findings in therapies for Burkitt lymphoma

The above items in points i to xiv above were described and discussed under the various heading below.

Etiology/Causes of BL

The exact cause of BL is not known. However, the lymphomas are characterized by a translocation and deregulation of a gene (c-myc) on chromosome 8 [10]. In addition, there has been an association between BL and a high incidence of malaria and/or infection with EBV [11-15]. Again, patients with a depressed immune response have also been noted to have a higher incidence of BL [6, 15, 16].

The etiological role of viral infection is supported by the finding that, in EBV-positive cases, every tumor cell has monoclonal EBV genomes [13, 16]. More research is required regarding the precise details of BL pathogenesis, specifically in terms of the nature of the B-cell initially infected with EBV, whether EBV infection precedes or follows the c-MYC translocation, and which viral genes are involved at different stages of the tumor transformation process [10, 13, 16].

Types of BL

The various types of BL are described below [11-19]:

Endemic BL

Endemic BL originates is Africa. It is the most common type of BL and the most common childhood cancer overall. It has an incidence rate of about 50 times higher in equatorial Africa and New Guinea than in the United States of America (USA). The most common site of endemic disease is the jaw. EBV has been shown to be linked to the endemic form of BL.

Sporadic BL

Sporadic BL occurs throughout the world. This form seen in the USA and Western Europe accounts for less than one percent of B-cell NHLs in adults; however, it accounts for 30% of all childhood lymphomas. An abdominal tumor is the most common site of disease occurrence.

Immunodeficiency-Related BL

Immunodeficiency-related variety of BL is most common in people with HIV/AIDS. It can also occur in patients who have inherited immune deficiencies or those who take immunosuppressive medications to prevent rejection after an organ transplant.

Epidemiology of BL

BL is a cancer of the lymphatic system that has significantly high incidence in equatorial Africa among children aged three to 16 years [11, 12, 17, 19]. The disease is characterized by tumors of the jaw bones and abdomen and is named after Denis Burkitt, who mapped is peculiar geographic distribution across Africa in the 1950s [2, 11, 12, 17, 19].

The EBV, which causes infectious mononucleosis, is present in most people suffering with BL [13, 17, 19]. However, this cancer is occasionally seen in areas of the world where it is not associated with the virus [16, 17, 19]. BL occurs more readily in people who have been weakened by malaria and in people suffering from AIDS [6, 16, 17, 19].

BL comprise about 1% to 2% of all lymphomas [5, 16, 17, 19]. The African variant of BL usually starts as a jaw tumor while in the USA, they usually begin as an abdominal tumor [16, 18, 19]. About 90% of these lymphomas occur in males [5, 18, 19]. In Africa, they occur mainly in children while in USA, the average age of onset is 30 years [5, 11, 12, 16, 18, 19].

Clinical Presentations of BL

As BL is highly aggressive, patients usually present with enlarged masses and signs of tumor lysis syndrome, with significantly elevated serum LDH and Ki-67 staining up to 95% [10, 18, 19]. Bone marrow and Central Nervous System (CNS) involvement can be found in 15%-30% of all cases [5, 12, 16, 18, 19]. Sporadic BL patients generally present with abdominal involvement, white endemic BL patients present with intra-oral masses, such as of the jaw or maxilla [11 – 19]. Immunodeficiency-associated BL is primarily seen in patients who are HIV-positive, particularly in those with low CD4 counts [6, 18, 19]. The clinical presentation includes CNS involvement or peripheral blood and bone marrow involvement [11-15, 18, 19].

Signs and symptoms of BL are somewhat in all types and may include the following [1, 2, 11-15, 18, 19]:

- nausea and vomiting
- loss of appetite
- abdominal pain
- abdominal masses in the jaw
- renal failure
- headaches
- visual impairment
- paraplegia
- night sweats
- weight loss
- fatigue
- enlarged lymph nodes
- gastrointestinal bleeding
- intestinal perforation

Abdominal symptoms are more prominent with BL seen in the USA, while endemic (African) BL tends to cause more jaw-related symptoms [1, 2, 11-15, 18, 19].

Clinical Evaluations of BL

The clinical evaluation of BL is always an emergency procedure. Bone marrow aspiration and biopsy and lumbar puncture are necessary to diagnose BL, in addition to liver and renal function tests and radiographic staging with Computed Tomography (CT) scan and Positron Emission Tomography (PET) of the chest, pelvis, and abdomen. The Ann Arbor staging system for the extent of disease evaluation is currently widely used [17-20]. In recent years, however, the Lugano classification has emerged as a useful tool for staging of NHL [17 – 20].

EBV and BL

EBV is a virus that is constantly part of the γ herpes virus subgroup/family which is widely accepted as having oncogenic viruses that expressed cancer genes and keeping infected-lymphocytes alive [13, 20]. EBV is the dominant viral infection in people, with about 95% of the global population exposed to it [13, 19, 20]. EBV is usually asymptomatic initially, but it can also present as mononucleosis. For many years, EBV has also been detected in cultured cells from BL patients, but it is also observed that EBV is not wholly critical in BL development and can also occur in its absence [13, 16, 20]. In addition, it is noted that the causative function of viral infection is supported by the observation that each cancer cell has monoclonal EBV genomes in EBV positive cases [16, 20]. Extra investigation is needed about the specific details of BL pathogenesis, particularly in terms of the nature of the B – cell firstly infected with EBV, and if EBV infection proceeds the c-MYC translocation, and which viral genes are involved at different stages of the cancer transformation process [10, 13, 20].

Diagnosis of BL

Diagnosis of BL depends upon pathologic evaluation of the involved tissue; consequently a bone marrow biopsy or aspiration is sometimes required and/or a tissue sample (for example, lymph node biopsy or a jaw tissue mass biopsy is done.). In addition to the biopsy, laboratory testing is usually done and imaging studies such as CT scanning and echocardiography would help in determining the extent of the disease. Other procedures or studies that may be performed are removal of fluid collections in the abdomen or thorax for cytogenetic evaluation.

Determination of the Staging of BL

The stage of a tumor is the extent to which it has spread in the body. Consequently, different researchers have different ways of staging BL [17-20]. For example, the National Cancer Institute (NCI) in the USA has a five stage system, which is as follows [19, 20]:

- A: Single solitary extra-abdominal site
- AR: Intra-abdominal, more than 90% of tumor resected
- B: Multiple extra-abdominal tumors
- C: Intra-abdominal tumor
- D: Intra-abdominal plus 1 or more extra-abdominal sites

The Michigan Ann Arbor system and St. Jude/Murphy system uses the following stages [21, 22]:

- Stage I: Single tumor (extranodal or outside a lymph node) or single anatomic area
- Stage II: Single tumor (extranodal) with regional node involved, primary gastrointestinal tumor and/or lymphoma involving nodal areas on the same side of the diaphragm
- Stage III: Lymphoma involving sites on opposite sides of the diaphragm, all primary intrathoracic tumors, all paraspinal or epidural tumors, and/or extensive intra-abdominal disease

It is therefore important for clinicians to discuss the staging system they are using with their patients in order to make informed decisions for better clinical outcomes.

Histology/Morphology and Cytogenetics

BL tumor cells are usually monomorphic with very limited pleomorphism. Importantly, the diagnosis of BL demonstrates cytogenetic characteristics of t(8;14) (q24:q32) and its variant translocation t(2;8) (p12:q24) and t(8;22) (q24;q11), occurring in 90% of cases, or c-MYC rearrangement [12, 23, 24]. The rate of Ki-67 proliferative index is usually >90%, and up to 100% in BL [23, 24]. However, a high Ki-67 by itself does not equate with BL [24]. Therefore, when diagnosing BL, karyotyping and FISH are commonly used to detect MYC translocation [24, 25].

Immunophenotype and Molecular Signature

BL is a subtype of B-cell NHL, for which positive B-cell markers are typically detected, including CD10, CD19, CD20, CD22, AND CD79a; BCL6 and monotypic surface IgM with kappa and lambda [18-20, 23-25]. BL cells do not usually express CD5 and CD23 or Terminal deoxynucleotidyl Transferase (TdT). Meanwhile, BCL2 is negative in most patients [19, 25]. The over proliferation of B-cells derived from the lymphoid cells' Germinal Center (GC) are separated into blast (centroblast) and centrocyte [22, 25]. The somatic hypermutation express immunoglobulin gene variable (IgV) region transform B-cells into neoplasm with either BL or diffuses Large B-Cell Lymphoma (DLBCL) [4, 23-25].

Treatment Choices for BL

Treatment of BL must be started promptly (ideally within 48 hours after diagnosis) including the prevention of Tumor Lysis Syndrome (TLS) [26, 27]. The unavoidable first step of treatment is the application of the prophase, with low-dose cyclophosphamide and prednisone [25-27]. This pre-phase helps to limit the risk of TLS by decreasing the release of cytokines, particularly in case of high tumor burden-a situation that can be lethal given the aggressiveness and chemo-sensitivity of the tumor burden [26, 27.]

The anti-CD20 monoclonal antibody rituximab transforms the management of other manure B-cell malignancies [27 – 29]. Clinical trials have demonstrated that adding rituximab to chemotherapy can improve patients' Overall Survival (OS). An efficacy benefit has also been shown in patients with BL and other aggressive lymphomas [28, 29]. However, in pediatrics, rituximab is given prior to chemotherapy [29]. As BL expresses CD20 positive markers in their cell surfaces, rituximab has been shown to improve the survival rate in this disease [30 – 36].

Furthermore, chemotherapy is the main treatment for BL [34-36]. Targeted therapy and CNS prophylaxis, including other treatment options like hematopoietic stem cell transplantation (HSCT) and immunotherapy and experimental agents may also be given. The description of each of the treatment options for BL is stated below.

Chemotherapy

Due to the aggressive nature of BL, diagnosis and workup should be completed as soon as possible to begin chemotherapy. Interestingly, different types of chemotherapy protocols are recommended, and the prognosis for this disease is good [35, 36]. The combinations of chemotherapy drugs that may be used to treat Burkitt lymphoma include [37 – 41]:

- CODOX-M – cyclophosphamide (Cytoxan, Procytox), vincristine (Oncovin), doxorubicin (Adriamycin) and high-dose methotrexate
- CODOX-M/IVAC (Magrath protocol) – CODOX-M plus IVAC, which is ifosfamide (Ifex), etoposide (Vepesid) and cytarabine (Cytosar, Ara-C)

- hyperCVAD – cyclophosphamide, vincristine, doxorubicin, dexamethasone (Decadron, Dexasone), methotrexate and cytarabine
- EPOCH – etoposide, prednisone, vincristine, cyclophosphamide and doxorubicin

As stated previously, TLS is a group of side effects that develops when a large number of lymphoma cells are killed in a short period of time [26, 27, 40, 41]. It often develops with chemotherapy for BL, so the healthcare team should take measures to prevent TLS before chemotherapy starts [26, 39, 40, 41].

Targeted Therapy

Targeted therapy uses drugs to target specific molecules (such as proteins) on the surface of cancer cells [37, 39, 40, 41]. These molecules help to send signals that tell cells to grow or divide [37, 40, 41]. By targeting these molecules, the drugs stop the growth and spread of cancer cells while limiting harm to normal cells [37, 38, 40, 41].

Rituximab (Rituxan, Truxima, Mabthera) is the most common targeted therapy used to treat BL [38, 40, 41]. It may be added to any of the above combinations of chemotherapy [38 – 41].

Central Nervous System Prophylaxis

CNS prophylaxis is used to try to prevent the lymphoma cells from entering the tissue covering the brain and spinal cord [30, 40, 41].

Methotrexate and cytarabine are used for CNS prophylaxis [41]. They are given as intrathecal chemotherapy. This means that they are injected into the cerebrospinal fluid (CSF) [30, 41].

High-dose methotrexate is also used for CNS prophylaxis [41]. It is given by a needle in a vein (intravenously) [40, 41].

Furthermore, other progresses in the treatments of BL are described and discussed as follows:

Progress on the Role of HSCT in the Treatment of BL

As BL may be cured through combination therapy, the use of HSCT has now decreased. Previous studies have evaluated HSCT in patients with BL [29-39, 42]. It has also been reported that a group of 117 patients who received autologous stem cell transplantation (SCT) in 1984 and 1994 showed a 72% 3-year overall survival (OS) for those in first time complete response to treatment (CR) [39 - 42].

Moreover, 37% of patients exhibited a chemotherapysensitive disease, but only 7% had a chemotherapy-resistant disease (retrospective analysis) [40, 42]. It has been argued that HSCT currently has no advantage in BL therapy compared to modern treatment regimens, and that it has no proven value for BL management [42 – 44]. The *'Hemato-Oncologie voor Volwassenen Nederland'* (HOVON – the Heamato Oncology Foundation for Adults in the Netherlands) group examined 27 patients, first using CR with initial dose chemotherapy, including two cycles of cyclophosphamide, doxorubicin, etoposide, mitoxantrone, and prednisone [40 - 44]. This was followed by autologous HCT and BEAM conditioning (carmustine, etoposide, cytarabine, melphalan). A five-years EFS was 73% and estimates OS of 81%, respectively [35, 40, 42-44].

Progress on Exploring the Use of Immunotherapy and Experimental Agents in the Treatment of BL

The various progresses on exploring the use of immunotherapy and experimental agents in the treatment of BL as described as follows:

The Effect of Ofatumumab and Obinutuzumab GA101

The development of B-cell lymphoid malignancy treatment has increased in recent years [42 – 45]. Several groups have increased the use of chemotherapy regimens and immunotherapy is also considered an acceptable choice [41 -45].

As BL cells express specific target markers, such as CD19, CD20, CD22 or CD52, much has been written about the improvement of anti-CD20 monoclonal antibodies (such as rituximab) in patients with BL [42, 45]. However, BL patients have also exhibited resistance to rituximab [45]. New studies have thus utilized other CD20-targeting agents, such as ofatumumab and obinutuzumab (GA101) [42 – 45].

Ofatumumab is a second-generation anti-CD20 monoclonal antibody that sticks to a site and is more effective than rituximab in inducing both cell-mediated and Complement-Dependent Cytotoxicity (CDC) [42, 45]. It works by targeting a membrane proximal small-loop epitope on the CD20 molecule [45]. Some studies have shown the effects of ofatumumab in Acute Lymphoblastic Leukemia (ALL) patients, for which promising CD20-positive results were achieved [46, 47].

Obinutuzumab is another type of glycoengineered humanized anti-CD20 antibody that has developed potency in B-cell malignancies and has been approved by the FDA for the upfront treatment of Chronic Lymphocytic Leukemia (CLL) [42, 45, 47]. Obinutuzumab is more effective than other CD-20 monoclonal antibodies due its ability to directly induce cell death. Some studies have reported finding promising preclinical results in ALL cell lines and xenograft, but thus far, no evidence has been found in clinical studies for ALL patients [42, 45, 47]. A preclinical trial developed has been by Awasthi et al. for children and adolescents, which involves rituximab resistant-BL and pre- ALL evaluation of atumumab- and Obinutuzumab-enhanced cell death against BL and pre-ALL [45 – 47].

Chimeric Antigen Receptor (CAR T-Cell)

Recent studies have demonstrated that clinical trials of an anti-CD19 chimeric antigen receptor CAR T-cell therapy aimed at fighting B-cell lymphoid malignancies, such as CLL and DLBCL [47 – 50] are being undertaken. This new technology uses gene-modified autologous T- cells with a CD19 antigen specificity that is mainly expressed on the surface of B-cells [48 – 50]. Therefore, this approach would be used in BL to improve treatment of advanced or Minimal Residual Disease (MRD) [49, 50]. New clinical trials have demonstrated that CAT-T cells can induce complete remission in a patient with refractory BL [51].

Immune-Checkpoint (PD-1 – PD-L1)

Other highly effective inhibitors for B-cell malignancies are programmed cell-death protein 1 (PD-1)/programmed cell death 1 ligand 1 (PD-L1) immune checkpoint inhibitors [51, 52]. These are the proteins that regulate immune cell activation to maintain self-tolerance and to prevent autoimmunity [52]. Interestingly, these proteins play an important role in controlling T-lymphocyte priming and activation.

Several studies have reported on the clinical benefits of the PD-1/PDL1 antibody in Follicular Lymphoma (FL) patients and DLBCL, as well as Hodgkin Lymphoma (HL) patients treated with nivolumab [53 – 56]. Other studies have reported that PD-1/PD-L1 are not expressed in BL cells, and hence PD-1/PD-L1 checkpoint inhibitors have not been demonstrated for BL [57, 58].

Some projects have further demonstrated that the EBV-Latent Membrane Protein (LMP) can also stimulate PD-L1 expression via AP-1 and JAK-STAT pathways in HL cells with diploids 9p24.1 in both EBV positive and -negative patients because the spreading of genetic alteration is similar, even though EBV-positive patients are more likely to have greater PD-L1 Immunohistochemistry (IHC) staining scores [55, 59].

An ongoing clinical trial was developed using CD19 CAR- T cells and PD-1 knockout engineered T-cells (CD19 CAR and PD-1 knockout engineered T-cell) in patients who exhibit a high risk of relapsed CD19 positive ALL+BL, and thus receive the CD19 CAR and PD-1 knockout engineered T-cell following lymphodepleting chemotherapy [58, 59]. This clinical trial demonstrates the safety, efficacy, and duration response of the CD19 CAR and PD-1 knockout engineered T-cells in patients with a high risk of relapsed CD19 positive malignancies [57 – 59].

Future Directions in MYC Inhibition

Due to the fact that majority of BL patients have an over-expression of the pathogenic MYC proto-oncogene, new experimental biologically targeted agents should be studied, particularly in patients with high-risk and relapsed refractory disease [60]. Direct and indirect MYC inhibitors are, therefore, particularly indicated in this aspect [10, 60].

Pharmacologic inhibition of MYC is difficult to achieve because of its several functions and targets [10, 59, 60]. Direct inhibitors, such as JQI and THZ1 that target MYC interactions may be useful in this regard 10, 60]. Interestingly, the link between JQI and MYC may also be involved in the dependence of MYC on bromodomain and Bromodomain Extraterminal Inhibitors (BET) protein BRD443 in combination with the PI3K pathway [10, 60 – 63].

Experimental studies have shown that mechanistically, the Mammalian Target of Rapamycin (MTOR) or Histone Deacetylase (HDAC) inhibitors may cause tumor regression [61 – 63]. Moreover, MTOR signaling plays an important role in tumor cell growth and is aberrantly activated in lymphoma [64, 65]. Several studies have demonstrated the effectiveness of unique combinations of the HDAC+MTOR and HDAC+BET inhibitors or BL/leukemia, therefore providing us with a new direction by targeting MYC proto-oncogene and associated proteins [66].

Progress on New Finding Therapies for BL

With newly developed technologies and advances in techniques, new drugs have been discovered that could undergo preclinical sensitivity screening using ex-vivo culture methods, with simultaneous testing for leukemia/lymphoma [67]. Related to B-cell lymphoid malignancies, some studies have shown venetoclax to be synergistic with vincristine and dexamethasone in B-precussor ALL expressing TCF3-HLF gene rearrangement [67, 68].

Recently, published studies have unveiled sets of additional recurrently mutated genes in B-cell malignancy patients (ID3, TCF3, and CCND3 occur in BL) [67 – 69]. Another study has demonstrated that birinapant, a SMAC mimetic inducer of apoptosis and necroptosis, was found to more effective against highly MRD-resistant patients of B-cell lineage ALL [68, 69].

PROGNOSIS OF THERAPIES

BL is rapidly progressive and universally fatal in the absence of therapy [35, 69]. In patients able to tolerate a dose-intensive chemotherapy program, timely initiation and completion of therapy can result in long-term survival [35, 36, 40, 69]. While most Patients will initially respond to treatment, progression-free and overall survival rates in adults have not matched outcomes in younger patients [39, 40, 69].

Investigators have reported two-year overall survival ranging from 67-92% in using the CODOX-M/IVAC regimen [37, 38, 69]. At five years, CALGB 9251 resulted in 52% of patients being alive and in complete remission [37, 38, 39, 60].

Three-year overall survival for hyper-CVAD has ranged from 49-89% [7, 69]. Six-year overall survival for DA-EPOCH-R has been reported to be 100%, albeit in 19 patients having a median age of 33 years [7, 68, 69]. For patients who relapse after initial therapy, salvage options should be considered, palliative care should be given to few patients achieving long-term survival.

CONCLUSION

BL is an uncommon and highly aggressive form of lymphoma. In the modern era, however, treatment with intensive and different combinations of chemo-immunotherapy can achieve excellent results. Nevertheless, in some relapsed/refractory patients, the prognosis remains poor. Most patients do not achieve second remission despite an intensive salvage treatment, and therefore urgent therapies are required to treat these patients. Several drugs that are currently undergoing clinical trials may provide new ways of treating BL. Evidence from our various searches show that our current work is the most up to date that discusses the advances in therapeutic measures for BL. Our future work will involve looking into more innovative ways of making fast diagnosis and timely treatments for BL in order to maximize efficient patient care and better prognosis and outcomes for sufferers of BL and their families.

REFERENCES

[1] Molyneux, E. M., Rochford, R., Griffin, B., Newton, R., Jackson, R., Menon, G., et al. (2012). Burkitt's lymphoma. *Lancet*, *379*, (9822), 1234-44.

[2] Burkitt, D. (1958). "A sarcoma involving the jaws in African children". *The British Journal of Surgery*, *46* (197), 218-23.

[3] O'Conor, G. T. & Davies, J. N. (1960). Malignant Tumors in African children. With special reference to malignant lymphoma. *J Pediatr.*, *56*, 526-535.

[4] Orem, J., Mbidde, E. K., Lambert, B., Sanjose, S. & Weiderpass, E. (2007). Burkitt's lymphoma in Africa, a review of the epidemiology and etiology. *Afr Health Sci.*, *7* (3), 166-175.

[5] Cardy, H. A., Sharp, L. & Little, J. (2001). Burkitt's lymphoma: a review of the epidemiology. *Kuwait med J.*, *33*, 293-306.

[6] Davi, F., Delecluse, H. J., Guiet, P., et al. (1998). Burkitt-like lymphomas in AIDS patients: characterization within a series of 103 human immunodeficiency virus-associated non-Hodgkin's lymphomas. Burkitt's Lymphoma Study Group. *J Clin Oncol.*, *16*(12), 3788-95.

[7] Thomas, D. A., Faderl, S., O'Brien, S., et al. (2006). Chemoimmunotherapy with hyper-CVAD plus rituximab for the treatment of adult Burkitt and Burkitt-type lymphoma or acute lymphoblastic leukemia. *Cancer*, *106*(7), 1569-80.

[8] Magrath, I., Adde, M., Shad, A., et al. (1996). Adults and children with small non-cleaved-cell lymphoma have a similar excellent outcome when treated with the same chemotherapy regimen. *J Clin Oncol.*, *14*(03), 925-34.

[9] Kantarjian, H. M., Walters, R. S., Keating, M. J., et al. (1990). Results of the vincristine, doxorubicin, and dexamethasone regimen in adults with standard- and high-risk acute lymphocytic leukemia. *J Clin Oncol.*, *8*(6), 994-1004.

[10] Dang, C. V., Resar, L. M., Emison, E., et al. (1999). Function of the c-Myc oncogenic transcription factor. *Exp Cell Res.*, *253*(1), 63-77.

[11] Burkitt, D. P. (1972). Classics in oncology. A sarcoma involving the jaws in African children. *CA Cancer J Clin.*, *22*(6), 345-55.

[12] Burkitt, D. & O'Conor, G. T. (1961). Malignant lymphoma in African children. I. A clinical syndrome. *Cancer*, *14*, 258-69.

[13] Epstein, M. A., Achong, B. G. & Barr, Y. M. (1964). Virus particles in cultured lymphoblast from Burkitt's lymphoma. *Lancet*, *1*(7335), 702-3.

[14] Magrath, I. (1990). The pathogenesis is Burkitt's lymphoma. *Adv Cancer Res.*, *55*, 133-270.

[15] Magrath, I. T. (1991). African Burkitt's lymphoma. History, biology, clinical features, and treatment. *Am J Pediatr Hematol Oncol.*, *13*(2), 222-46.

[16] Magrath, I. (2012). Epidemiology: Clues to the pathogenesis of Burkitt lymphoma. *Br J Haematol.*, *56*(6), 744-756.

[17] Swerdlow, S. H., Campo, E., Pileri, S. A., Harris, N. L., Stein, H., Siebert, R., et al. (2016). The 2016 revision of the World Health Organization classification of lymphoid neoplasms. *Blood*, *127* (20), 2375-90.

[18] Campo, E., Swerdlow, S. H., Harris, N. L., Pileri, S., Stein, H. & Jaffe, E. S. (2011). The 2008 WHO classification of lymphoid

neoplasms and beyond: evolving concepts and practical applications. *Blood*, *117*(19), 5019-5032.

[19] Cheson, B. D., Fisher, R. I., Barrington, S. F., Cavalli, F., Schwartz, L. H., Zucca, E., et al. (2018). Recommendations for Initial Evaluation, Staging, and Response Assessment of Hodgkin and Non-Hodgkin lymphoma: The Lugano Classification. *J Clin Oncol.*, *32*(27), 3059-3068.

[20] Standlund, J. T. (2012). Burkitt lymphoma: staging and response evalution. *Br J Haematol.*, *156*(6), 761-5.

[21] https://radiopaedia.org/articles/ann-arbor-staging-system Accessed on 16 May 2021.

[22] https://www.researchgate.net/figure/Murphy-St-Judes-staging-system-32_fig1_6135606 Accessed on 16 May 2021.

[23] Bertrand, S., Berger, R., Philip, T., Bernheim, A., Bryon, P. A., Bertoglio, J., et al. (1981). Variant translocation in a non-endemic case of Burkitt's lymphoma: t(8;22) in an Epstein-Barr virus negative tumour and in a derived cell line. *Eur J Cancer*, *17*(5), 577-581.

[24] Bernheim, A., Berger, R. & Legior, G. (1981). Cytogenetic Studies on African Burkitt's Lymphoma Cell Linesa ¯:t(8;14), t(2;8) and t(8;22) Translocations. *Cancer Genet Cytogenet*, *3*(4), 307-315.

[25] Abate, F., Ambrosio, M. R., Mundo, L., Laginestra, M. A., Fuligni, F., Rossi, M., et al. (2015). Distinct Viral and Mutational Spectrum of Endemic Burkitt Lymphoma. *PLoS Pathog.*, *11*(10), 1-21.

[26] Cairo, M. S. & Bishop, M. (2004). Tumour lysis syndrome: new therapeutic strategies and classification. *Br J Haematol*, *127*(1), 3-11.

[27] Barnes, J. A., LaCasce, A. S., Feng, Y., Toomey, C. E., Neuberg, D., Michaelson, J. S., et al. (2011). Evaluation of the addition of rituximab to CODOX-M/IVAC for Burkitt's lymphoma: A retrospective analysis. *Ann Oncol.*, *22*(8), 1859-1864.

[28] Corazzelli, G., Frigeri, F., Russo, F., Frairia, C., Arcamone, M., Esposito, G., et al. (2011). RD- CODOX-M/IVAC with rituximab and intrathecal liposomal cytarabine in adult Burkitt lymphoma and 'unclassifiable' highly aggressive B-cell lymphoma. *Br J Haematol.*, *156*(2), 234-244.

[29] Evens, A. M., Carson, K. R., Kolesar, J., Nabhan, C., Helenowski, I., Islam, N., et al. (2013). A multicenter phase II study incorporating high-dose rituximab and liposomal doxorubicin into the CODOX-M/IVAC regimen for untreated Burkitt's lymphoma. *Ann Oncol.*, *24*(12), 3076-3081.

[30] Thomas, D. A., Cortes, J., O'Brien, S., Pierce, S., Faderl, S., Albitar, M., et al. (1999). Hyper- CVAD program in Burkitt's-type adult acute lymphoblastic leukemia. *J Clin Oncol.*, *17*(8), 2461-2470.

[31] Thomas, D. A., Faderl, S., O'Brien, S., Ramos, B. C., Cortes, J., Garcia-Manero, G., et al. (2006). Chemoimmunotherapy with hyper-CVAD plus rituximab for the treatment of adult Burkitt and Burkitt-type lymphoma or acute lymphoblastic leukemia. *Cancer*, *106*(7), 1569-1580.

[32] Magrath, I., Adde, M., Shad, A., Venzon, D., Seibel, N., Gootenberg, J., et al. (1996). Adults and children with small non-cleaved-cell lymphoma have a similar excellent outcome when treated with the same chemotherapy regimen. *J Clin Oncol.*, *14*(3), 925-934.

[33] Rizzeri, D. A., Johnson, J. L., Niedzwiecki, D., Lee, E. J., Vardiman, J. W., Powell, B. L., et al. (2004). Intensive Chemotherapy with and without Cranial Radiation for Burkitt Leukemia and Lymphoma Final Results of Cancer and Leukemia Group B Study 9251. *Cancer*, *100*(7), 1438-1448.

[34] Intermesoli, T., Rambaldi, A., Rossi, G., Delaini, F., Romani, C., Pogliani, E. M., et al. (2013). High cure rates in Burkitt lymphoma and leukemia: a Northern Italy Leukemia Group study of the German short intensive rituximab-chemotherapy program. *Haematologica*, *98*(11), 1718-1725.

[35] Rizzeri, D. A., Johnson, J. L., Byrd, J. C., Lozanski, G., Blum, K. A., Powell, B. L., et al. (2014). Improved efficacy using rituximab and brief duration, high intensity chemotherapy with filgrastim support for Burkitt or aggressive lymphomas: Cancer and Leukemia Group B study 10 002. *Br J Haematol.*, *165*(1), 102- 111.

[36] Dunleavy, K., Pittaluga, S., Shovlin, M., Steinberg, S. M., Cole, D., Grant, C., et al. (2013). Low-Intensity Therapy in Adults with Burkitt's Lymphoma. *N Engl J Med.*, *369*(20), 1915-1925.

[37] Mead, G. M., Sydes, N. R., Walewski, J., Grigg, A., Hatton, C. S., Pescosta, N., Guarnaccia, C., Lewis, M. S., McKendrick, J., Stenning, S. P., Wright, D. & Norbert, P. (2002). UKLG LY06 collaborators. An international evaluation of CODOX-M and CODOX-M alternating with IVAC in Adult Burkitt's lymphoma: results of United Kingdom Lymphoma Group LY06 study. *Ann Oncol.*, *13*(8), 1264-74.

[38] Barnes, J. A., Lacasce, A. S., Feng, Y., Toomey, C. E., Neuberg, D. & Michaelson, J. S. (2011). Hochberg EP, Abramson JS, Evaluation of the addition of rituximab to CODOX-M/IVAC for Burkitt's lymphoma: a retrospective analysis. *Ann Oncol.*, *22*(8), 1859-64.

[39] Thomas, D. A., Faderl, S., O'Brien, S., Bueso-Ramos, C., Cortes, J., Garcia-Monero, G., Giles, F. J., Verstovsek, S., Wierda, W. G., Pierce, S. A., Shan, J., Brandt, M., Hagemeister, F. B., Keating, M. J., Cabanillas, F. & Kantarjian, H. (2006). Chemoimmunotherapy with hyper-CVAD plus rituximab for the treatment of adult Burkitt and Burkitt-type lymphoma or acute lymphoblastic leukemia. *Cancer*, *106*(7), 1569-80.

[40] Dunleavy, K., Pittaluga, S., Shovlin, M., Steinberg, S. M., Cole, D., Gtant, C., Widemann, B., Staudt, L. M., Jaffe, E. S., Little, R. F. & Wilson, W. H. (2013). (Low-intensity therapy in adults with Burkitt's lymphoma. *N Engl J Med.*, *369*(20), 1915-25.

[41] *Burkitt lymphoma.* https://www.cancer.ca/en/cancer-information/cancer-type/non-hodgkin-lymphoma/non-hodgkin-lymphoma/more-types-of-nhl/burkitt-lymphoma/?region=on. Accessed on May 16 2021.

[42] Intermesoli, T., Rambaldi, A., Rossi, G., Delaini, F., Romani, C., Pogliani, E. M., et al. (2013). High cure rates in Burkitt lymphoma and leukemia: a Northern Italy Leukemia Group study of the German short insensitive rituximab-chemotherapy program. *Haematologica.*, *98*(11), 1718-1725.

[43] Sweetenham, B. J. W., Pearce, R., Taghipour, G., Blaise, D., Gisselbrecht, C. & Goldstone, A. H. (2018). Adult Burkitt's and Burkitt-like Non-Hodgkin's Lymphoma-Outcome for Patients Treated With High-Dose Therapy and Autologous Stem-Cell Transplantation in First Remission or at Relapse: Results From the European Group for Blood and Marrow Transplantation. *J Clin Oncol.*, *14*(9), 2465-2472.

[44] Imhoff, G. W. V., Holt, B. V. D., Mackenzie, M. A., Ossenkoppele, G. J., Wijermasn, P. W., Kramer, M. H., et al. (2005). Short intensive sequential therapy followed by autologous stem cell transplantation in adult Burkitt, Burkitt'-like and lymphoblastic lymphoma, *Leukemia.*, *19*(6), 945-952.

[45] Awasthi, A., Ayello, J., Ven, C. V. D., Elmacken, M., Sabulski, A., Barth, M. J., et al. (2015). Obinutuzumab (GA101) compared to rituximab significantly enhances cell death and antibody-dependent cytotoxicity and improves overall survival against CD20(+) rituximab-sensitive/-resistant Burkitt lymphoma (BL) and precursor B- acute lymphoblastic leukemia (pre-B-ALL): potential targeted therapy in patients with poor risk CD20(+) BL and pre-B-ALL. *Br J Haematol.*, *17*(5), 1, 763-775.

[46] Tobinai, K., Klein, C., Oya, N. & Rowson, F. G. (2017). A Review of Obinutuzumab (GA101), a Novel Type II Anti-CD20 Monoclonal Antibody, for the Treatment of Patients with B-Cell Malignancies. *Abv Ther.*, *34*(2), 324-356.

[47] Porter, D. L., Levine, B. L., Kalos, M., Bagg, A. J. C. & June, C. H. (2011). Chimeric Antigen Receptor-Modified T Cells in Chronic Lymphoid Leukemia. *N Engl J Med.*, *365*(8), 1507-1517.

[48] Maude, S. L., Frey, N., Shaw, P. A., Aplenc, R., Barrett, D. M., Bunin, N. J., et al. (2014). Chimeric Antigen Receptor T Cells for Sustained Remissions in Leukemia. *N Engl Med.*, *371*(16), 1507-1517.

[49] Kochenderfer, J. N., Feldman, S. A., Zhao, Y., Xu, H., Black, M. A., Morgan, R. A., et al. (2010). Construction and Pre-clinical

Evaluation of an Anti-CD19 Chimeric Antigen Receptor. *J Immunother*, *32*(7), 689-702.

[50] Kochenderfer, J. N., Dudley, M. E., Kassim, S. H., Somerville, R. P. T., Carpenter, R. O., Stetler-Stevenson, M., et al. (2015). Chemotherapy-refractory diffuse large B-cell lymphoma and indolent B-cell malignancies can be effectively treated with autologous T cells expressing an anti-CD19 chimeric antigen receptor. *J Clin Oncol.*, *33*(6), 540-549.

[51] Antigdor, A., Shouval, R., Jacoby, E., Davidson, T., Shimoni, A., Besser, M., et al. (2018). CAR T cells induce a complete response in refractory Burkitt Lymphoma. *Bone Marrow Tranplant.*, *53*(12), 1583-1585.

[52] Goodman, A., Patel, S. P. & Kurzrock, R. (2017). PD-1-PD-L1 immune-checkpoint blockade in B-cell lymphomas. *Nat Rev Clin Oncol.*, *14*(4), 203-220.

[53] Westin, J. R., Chu, F., Zhang, M., Fayad, L. E., Fowler, N., Romaguera, J., et al. (2014). Safety and Activity of PD1 Blockade by Pidilizumab in Combination with Rituximab in Patients with Relapsed Follicular Lymphoma: a Single Group, Open-label, Phase 2 Trial. *Lancet Oncol.*, *15*(1), 69-77.

[54] Armand, P., Nagler, A., Weller, E. A., Devine, S. M., Avigan, D. E., Chen, Y. B., et al. (2013). Disabling immune tolerance by programmed death-1 blockade with pidilizumab after autologous hematopoietic stem-cell transplantation for diffuse large b-cell: Results of an International Phase II Trial. *Journal of Clinical Oncology*, *31*(33), 4199-4206.

[55] Roemer, M. G. M., Advani, R. H., Ligon, A. H., Natkunam, Y., Redd, R. A., Homer, H., et al. (2016). PD-L1 and PD-L2 genetic alterations define classical Hodgkin lymphoma and predict outcome. *J Clin Oncol.*, *34*(23), 2690-2697.

[56] Fowler, N. H., Cheah, C. Y., Gascoyne, R. D., Gribben, J., Neelapu, S. S., Ghia, P., et al. (2016). Role of the tumor microenvironment in mature B-cell lymphoid malignancies. *Haemotologica.*, *101*(5), 531-540.

[57] Andorsky, D. J., Yamada, R. E., Said, J., Pinkus, G. S., Betting, D. J., Timmerman, J. M., et al. (2011). Programmed death ligand 1 is expressed by non-Hodgkin lymphomas and inhibits the activity of tumor-associated T cells. *Clin Cancer Res.*, *17*(13), 4232-4244.

[58] Chen, B. J., Chapuy, B., Ouyang, J., Sun, H. H., Roemer, M. G. M., Hu, M. L., et al. (2012). PD-L1 expression is characteristic of a subset of aggressive B-cell lymphomas and virus-associated malignancies. *Clin Cancer Res.*, *18*(6), 1611-1618.

[59] Green, M. R., Rodig, S., Juszczynski, P., Ouyang, J., Sinha, P., O'Donnell, E., et al. (2012). Constitutive AP-1 activity and EBV infection induce PD-L1 in Hodgkin lymphomas and posttransplant lymphoproliferative disorders: Implications for targeted therapy. *Clin Cancer Res.*, *18*(6), 1611-1618.

[60] Blum, K. A., Lozanski, G. & Byrd, J. C. (2012). Adult Burkitt leukemia and lymphoma. *Blood.*, *104*, 3009-3020.

[61] Pasternak, V. & Cole, M. D. (2016). Strategically targeting MYC in cancer. *F100Research.*, *5*, 408.

[62] Anderson, M. A., Tsui, A., Wall, M., Huang, D. C. S. & Roberts, A. W. (2016). Current challenges and novel treatment strategies is double hit lymphomas. *Ther Adv Hematol*. 5:408.

[63] Hartl, M. The Quest for Targets Executing MYC-Dependent Cell Transformation. *Front Oncol.*, 2016, 6, 132.

[64] Hay, N. & Sonenberg, N. (2013). Cancer genomics: the post-transcriptional era. *Curr Opin Genet Dev.*, 23(1), 1-2.

[65] Witzig, T. E. & Gupta, M. (2010). Signal transduction inhibitor therapy for lymphoma. Hematology *Am Soc Hematol Educ Program.*, *8*, 265-270.

[66] Muralidharan, S. V., Bhadury, J., Nilsson, L. M., Green, L. C., McLure, K. G., Nilsson, J. A., et al. (2016). BET bromodomain inhibitors synergize with ATR inhibitors to induce DNA damage, apoptosis, senescence-associated secretory pathway and ER stress in Myc-induced lymphoma cells. *Oncogene.*, *35*(36), 4689-4697.

[67] Fischer, U., Forster, M., Rinaldi, A., Risch, T., Sungalee, S., Warnatz, H. J., et al. (2015). Genomics and drug profiling of fatal

TCF3-HLF- positive acute lymphoblastic leukemia identifies recurrent mutation patterns and therapeutic options. *Nat Genet.*, *47*(9), 1020-1029.

[68] McComb, S., Gorgorio, J. A., Harder, L., Marovca, B., Cario, G., Eckert, C., et al. (2016). Activation of concurrent apoptosis and necroptosis by SMAC minetics for the treatment of refractory and relapsed ALL. *Sci Transl Med.*, *8*(339), 339-370.

[69] Rohde, M., Bonn, B. R., Zimmermann, M., Large, J., Moricke, A., Klapper, W., et al. (2017). Relevance of ID3-TCF3-CCND3 pathway mutations in pediatric aggressive B-cell lymphoma treated according to the non-Hodgkin lymphoma Berlin-Frankfurt-munster protocols. *Haematologica.*, *102*(6), 1091-1098.

In: Burkitt Lymphoma
Editor: Douglas V. Berthelot
ISBN: 978-1-68507-071-7

Chapter 6

Burkitt Lymphoma: Evaluation of Characteristics, Clinical Updates and Management Approaches Trends

Daniella E.C.C.O.H Kingsley-Godwin*, MD, PhD,
Maria Jana Kingsley Godwin
and Joshua Kingsley-Godwin, PhD
London Medical Academy, London, England, United Kingdom

Abstract

Burkitt lymphoma is an uncommon but highly aggressive B-cell Non-Hodgkin Lymphoma. It is a subtype of mature B-cell lymphoma and can be treated successfully within a short period via high-intensity chemotherapeutic regimens. Diagnosis and initial workup must be completed rapidly to begin treatment due to high proliferation of the disease. Burkitt lymphoma is associated with the Epstein-Barr Virus and with chromosomal translocation that activates the c-MYC gene. However, by implementing chemotherapy regimens, complete remission

---

* Corresponding Author's E-mail: daniellagodwin@ymail.com and dkingsley@iahcp.uk.

and overall survival for young patients with BL remains high. In contrast, in elderly patients and those with relapsed/refractory disease, the prognosis remains a medical challenge. Rituximab has been shown to improve patient survival rate. However, because resistance can still occur, further treatment and evaluation is required, including inhibition of the MYC proto-oncogene through the use of bromodomain inhibitors. In this clinical systematic review and experts' opinions analysis, we explore and emphasise the trends and issues in research and innovation in the characteristics, clinical updates and management approaches of Burkitt lymphoma.

Keywords: Burkitt lymphoma, characteristics, clinical, updates, management, diagnosis, risk factors, epidemiology, treatment, etiology, chemotherapy, research, innovation, Epstein-Barr Virus, MYC, Non-Hodgkin

Introduction

Burkitt lymphoma (BL) is a type of mature B-cell non-Hodgkin lymphoma (NHL) [1]. Epstein- Barr virus (EBV) is a known risk factor, and most people diagnosed with Burkitt lymphoma are infected with this virus [1, 2]. Burkitt lymphoma can be divided into sporadic, endemic and immunodeficiency-related variants [2]. Thus, it is a very fast-growing (aggressive) type of NHL [3]. It tends to occur in organs or tissues other than the lymph nodes (called extranodal sites) [3]. It often spreads to the brain or spinal cord (called the central nervous system, or CNS) [1-3].

BL can affect the bone marrow so that it does not work normally [1, 2, 4]. As a result, blast cells don't mature properly, and these abnormal immature blood cells (called BL cells) are found in the circulating blood [1, 3, 4]. If more than 25% of the cells in the bone marrow are BLcells, doctors may classify it as acute lymphocytic leukemia (ALL), L3 or BL [1-3].

There is also a Burkitt-like lymphoma (BLL) [1, 3, 4]. When viewed under a microscope, BLL cells look somewhat different from BL cells.

They also have some features of diffuse large B-cell lymphoma (DLBCL) cells and as a result, BLL is grouped with BL [1, 4].

In addition, BL is a rapidly progressive lymphoma malignancy requiring a prompt diagnosis and administration of therapy. Often, therapy needs to be started before the results of molecular studies, which typically confirm the diagnosis [5]. A goal of initiating therapy within 48 hours of presentation has been proposed as optimal treatment for BL [2, 3, 5]. Therefore, a high degree of suspicion is required along with surgical colleagues who can rapidly obtain tissue for review by an expert haematopathologist [2-5]. The purpose of this clinical systematic review and experts' opinions analysis is to explore and emphasise the trends and issues in research and innovation in the characteristics, clinical updates management approaches of BL.

METHODS

Clinical systematic review and experts' opinions evaluation methods were used in carrying out this study. A literature search of characteristics, clinical updates and management approaches advances for BL was performed to locate publications and reports written in English language, using electronic databases such as of PubMed, EMBASE, SCOPUS, etc. form May 1954 to May 2021. The following search terms were input:

1. Burkitt lymphoma or Burkitt's lymphoma (Title/Abstract/full text).
2. Characteristics and clinical updates in Burkitt lymphoma (Title/Abstract/full text).
3. Management approaches of Burkitt lymphoma (Title/Abstract/full text).
4. Trends in research and innovations in Burkitt lymphoma (Title/Abstract/full text).

All of the authors of this article investigated all relevant studies for quality and publication date. Particularly, a list of references was added manually.

RESULTS

The searches yielded 2,035 published materials. After further review and refinements of the articles/publications, 41 references were selected to be used in conducting this study. The results of the findings from the terms stated in the "methods" section above were grouped under the following items:

(a) Etiology of BL
(b) Clinical Characteristics and Manifestations of BL
(c) Epidemiological Updates on BL
(d) Diagnosis Updates and Differential Diagnosis of BL
(e) Trends in the Management Approaches of BL
(f) Updates on Prognosis of BL

All the items stated in points (a) to (f) above are each described in the sections below.

Etiology of BL

In most cases BL is associated with a specific translocation t(8;14)(q23;q32) that juxtaposes the MYC/c-Myc gene (8q24) next to the heavy chain immunoglobulin gene (14q32) [6, 7]. In rare cases the translocation affects chromosome 2 (kappa chain in immunoglobulins) or 22 (lambda chain in immunoglobulins) [7, 8]. The cells express surface immunoglobulins and B differentiation markers (CD19, CD20) [6 -9]. The proliferation index of the tumor is extremely high (Ki67>95%) [4-9]. EBV influences the genesis of the endemic form of BL, but the mechanisms responsible are not well understood [6, 8, 9].

Clinical Characteristics and Manifestations

The characteristic feature of BL is a rapidly growing mass and elevated serum Lactate Dehydrogenase (LDH). Patients with the human immunodeficiency virus (HIV) in whom antiviral treatment is ineffective are particularly susceptible to BL [5, 7-9]. Two forms of the disease mostly exist in clinic: an `endemic' form (sub tropical Africa) linked to EBV that presents classically in the form of a maxillary tumor (an abdominal tumor is often present, particularly in older children), and a `sporadic' form not linked to EBV that develops mainly in the abdomen [6, 8-11]. The endemic variant of BL observed in equatorial Africa – a rapidly progressive jaw or orbital tumor – is the most common presentation, occurring more frequently in young children [5, 11-13]. In western countries where sporadic BL occurs more commonly, this presentation is relatively rare [10-13].

BL can also develop in the ear, nose and throat and more rarely in other locations (orbit, kidney bone) [4, 6, 11-13]. The tumor is very proliferative and secondarily invades the bone marrow (in about 35% of cases) and the central nervous system (in about 15% of cases) [6, 8, 9, 11, 13]. It has the appearance of tumoral meningitis or paralysis of the cranial nerves [3, 6, 8-13].

Abdominal disease can present with a variety of symptoms ranging from nausea, vomiting and a change in bowel habits to gastrointestinal bleeding and intestinal perforation [5, 8, 9, 13]. Extranodal disease is not uncommon, with numerous reports describing organ invasion, pleural effusions and ascites, as well as pharyngeal and sinus involvement [4, 9, 13].

Bone marrow involvement is documented in roughly 20% of cases of sporadic BL and may be much less common in the endemic variant [9, 10, 12, 13]. Central nervous system involvement has been reported in up to one-third of patients, is typically associated with other sites of extranodal involvement, and appears more frequently in endemic BL [8, 10, 11, 13].

Other NHL histologies need to be differentiated from BL [2-10]. Diffuse large B-cell lymphoma (DLBCL) is the most common NHL and may have a MYC rearrangement in 5% of cases [6-9, 13]. Given the relative incidence of DLBCL, BL occurs less commonly in developes countries than MYC+ DLBCL [6-9, 12, 13].

Cases with morphologic features intermediate between DLBCL and BL are called "B-cell lymphoma, unclassifiable, with features intermediate between DLBCL and BL" as per the current Word Health Organization (WHO) classification [14]. Differentiating these entities via expert hematopathologic review and appropriate molecular testing is critical given the major differences in treatments [9-14].

Other lymphoma histologies, including lymphoblastic lymphoma and blastic mantle cell lymphoma, present in a similar fashion to sporadic BL in adults [9-13, 15]. In younger patients, Wilms' tumor, neuroblastoma and soft tissue sarcomas should be considered in the differential diagnosis [16].

Burkitt leukemia, with the clinical characteristics of other types of leukemia, is possible [11, 13, 15, 16]. The tumors develop from the digestive tract (mainly the intestine) and extend to the peritoneum and sometimes it can be present in the liver, pancreas, spleen, kidneys or ovaries [11, 16]. The most frequent clinical signs and symptoms are abdominal pain, nausea, an alteration of general stare and/or other appearance of lymph nodes and tumors [11-16]. As can be seen in this sub-section, the characteristics and manifestations of BL are important factor in the disease and should be dealt with carefully in other to achieve a good outcome for the patient.

Epidemiological Updates

BL develops most often in children or young adults and is uncommon in older adults [16, 18]. It occurs most often in boys [18].

In developed countries where sporadic cases are most commonly encountered, BL can occur at any age, although the peak incidence is the first decade of life [16-18]. Roughly equal numbers of children and adults are affected [9, 11, 13, 18]. As such, BL accounts for 30%of pediatric lymphomas and less than 1% of lymphoma cases in adults [11-13, 15, 18]. The disease incidence is two to three time higher in equatorial Africa [10 – 18]. Termed endemic BL, the majority of cases are EBV-related [6, 7-13, 18]. The immunodeficiency related variant is most commonly associated with human immunodeficiency virus (HIV) infection, where one in three of cases are also EBV-related [19].

In Europe and North America it represents around half of all malignant non-Hodgkin lymphoma in children and around 2% in adults [20]. Two incidence peaks occur: one in childhood/adolescence and the second after the age of 40 years [20, 21]. Again, in Europe the standardized incidence ratio is 1/530,000 for individuals aged between 0 and 14 years and 1/670,000 for individuals aged between 15 and 19 years [20 – 22]. Males are affected more than females 19-22].

DIAGNOSIS UPDATES

Diagnosis is based on biopsy of a mass, an effusion puncture or bone marrow that reveals the presence of tumor cells [5, 6, 22]. The extent of the tumor can be evaluate using images (mainly ultrasound and scanning) [5, 22].

In most cases, the diagnosis is most readily made by an excisional lymph node biopsy [5, 23]. In cases where an excisional biopsy is difficult, multiple core needle biopsies may be adequate [5, 6, 23]. Expert hematopathologic review is essential.

The distinct starry-sky pattern of classic BL, (Figure 1) [23] in the setting of a histologic proliferative fraction approaching 100% may quickly suggest the diagnosis while variants that are more unusual may be harder to distinguish. The most commonly used measure of proliferation is the Ki-

67 [5, 23]. In BL, nearly 100% of the cells stains positive for Ki-67 [3, 5, 6, 23].

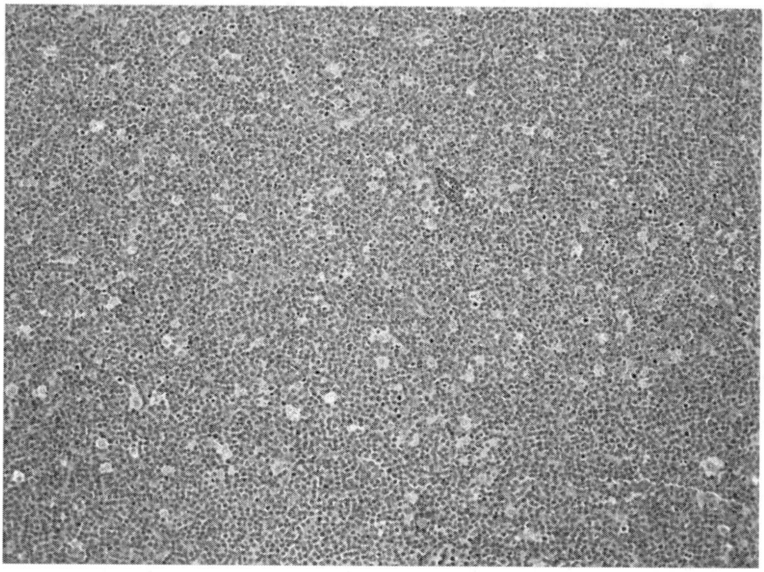

Figure 1. The "starry sky" appearance of BL characterized by benign macrophages interspersed among a diffuse infiltration of monotonous malignant lymphoctyes [23].

A translocation involving the MYC oncogene is identified in the majority of patients [7, 8, 23]. Classic BL demonstrates the t(8; 14)(q24;q32) reciprocal translocation involving the immunoglobulin heavy chain locus in 80% of cases [7-9, 19, 23]. Variants involving the light chain loci, t(8;22)(q24;q11) and t(2;8)(p12;q24), are less common [23].

Fluorescence *in situ* hybridization (FISH) to identify the MYC break-apart is routinely used along with routine karyotype analysis [7-9, 23]. Due to the molecular heterogeneity of chromosomal translocations causing MYC overexpression, polymerase chain reaction (PCR)-based testing to confirm their presence is not available [7, 9, 23]. While diffuse large B-cell lymphoma can also demonstrate a t (8; 14) translocation or MYC overexpression, this typically occurs in the context of other cytogenetic abnormalities [7-9, 20, 23].

Routine staging studies, including computed tomography of the neck, chest, abdomen, and pelvis +/- position emission tomography (PET), and bone marrow aspiration/biopsy, are indicated in the initial evaluation and ideally should be expedited so as not to delay therapy [5, 23].

The Ann Arbor staging system continues to be used in adult patients [24], however, some individual treatment regimens have been developed with individualized risk-adapted therapeutic plans. In addition, a serum lactate dehydrogenase is used in treatment planning [23, 24]. Routine laboratory testing should include an evaluation of renal and hepatic function as well as testing for HIV [19, 24]. A study of cardiac ejection fraction is necessary for patients who will receive anthracyclines as part of their treatment [5, 24]. A lumber puncture is indicated to exclude involvement of the cerebral spinal fluid [5, 20, 24]. Despite the presence or absence of neurologic symptoms, this is frequently performed in conjunction with intrathecal chemotherapy as systemic treatment is initiated [5, 25].

Differential Diagnosis

Differential diagnoses include other forms of abdominal tumors in children (Wilms tumor and neuroblastomas, although these are retroperitoneal, and desmoplastic tumors, including peripheral neuroectodermal tumors, including neuroblastoma and pediatric neuroblastoma) and other types of lymphoma and leukemia of B and T precursors in cases with bone marrow involvement [26]. Great difficulty is differentiate BL from diffuse large B-cell lymphoma (DLBCL), lymphoblastic lymphoma and blastic mantle cell lymphoma (MCL) among peripheral B-cell lymphomas [25, 26].

Other differential diagnoses of BL are acute lymphoblastic leukemia and follicular lymphoma and others.

Trends in the Management Approaches of BL

The rapid administration of chemotherapy, ideally within 48 hours of presentation, is of utmost importance in BL [27]. Aggressive hydration and recombinant urate oxidase (rasburicase) for hyperuricemia are currently recommended as prophylaxis against tumor lysis syndrome [28].

Therapy in general consists of dose-intense multi-agent chemotherapy regimen to provide additional time in completing the initial work-up as well as to further protect against tumor lysis syndrome and improve the patient's performance status [28, 29]. Based on many experience in pediatric patients, the most effective therapies for adult BL include chemotherapeutic agents administered in dose-intensive fashion as part of short duration regimens [30, 31]. In addition, the include agents such as methotrexate and cytrarabine which penetrate the central nervous system when administered in high doses as well as intrathecal prophylaxis or treatment [30-32]. Several regimens using similar agents have been reported [29-32]. On the basis of data available, a few may be preferable in adults. However, as demonstrated by retrospective analysis of 470 adult patients treated on prospective trails, inferior outcomes have been demonstrated in older patients (defined as >40 years in this series) [28 – 32]. Standard first-line regimens include [33-36]:

Table 1. Dose modified CODOX-M [36]

Cyclophosphamide 800 mg/m2IV on day 1
Cyclophosphamide 200 mg/m2IV od days 2-5
Doxorubicin 40 mg.m2IV on day 1
Vincristine 1.5 mg/m2(max 2 mg) on days 1 and 8
Methotrexate 300 mg/m2IV over 1 hour on day 10, then 2700 mg/m2IV given over next 23 hours. (For patients older than 65 years, 100 mg/m^2 is administered over 1 hour followed by 900 mg/m2over the next 23 hours). Leucovorin rescue begins 36 hours from the start of the methotrexate infusion.
Granulocyte colony-stimulating factor started on day 13and continues the absolute neutrophil count is > 1.0x109/L
Intrathecal prophylaxis:
Cytarabine 70 mg IT on days 1 and 3
Methotrexate 12 mg IT od days 15

Table 2. In IVAC [36]

Ifosfamide 1500 mg/m2IV on days 1-5 with mesna uroprotection
(For patients older than 65 years, dose of ifosfamide is 1000 mg/m2)
Etoposide 60 mg/m2IV od days 1-5
Cytarabine 2 g/m2IV every 12 hours on days 1 and 2 (4 doses)
(For patients older than 65 years, dose of cytarabine is 1 g/m2)
Granulocyte colony-stimulating factor begins on day 7 and continues
Until the absolute neutrophil count is > 1.0x109/L
Intrathecal prophylaxis:
Methotrexate 12 mg IT on day 5

1. Developed at the National Cancer Institute (NCI), this regimen uses the strategies described above and employs a two-group risk-stratification scheme base on Ann Arbor stage and lactate acid dehydrogenase (LHD). Patients with normal LHD, a performance status of 0-1 and stage 1-2 disease are defined as having low-risk disease and receive 3 cycles of CODOX-M [24, 33, 36]. All others are defined as having low risk disease and are treated with 4 alternating cycles of CODOX-M (Tables 1 and 2) [34, 36].
2. The regimen has been refined over several investigations for adult patients leading to reductions neurologic toxicity, myelosuppression, and mucosities [33, 36]. In turn, a two-year progression free survival of 64% has been reported in the three most recent investigations, albeit with the majority of patients studied being less than 40 years of age [34, 36]. Preliminary results demonstrate that incorporating the anti-CD 20 antibody rituximab does not increase toxicity [34 – 36]. Regimens developed by LMB and BFM groups are similar in the chemotherapeutics used, dose-intensity and risk adapted design [35, 36]. However, limited data is available for adults.
3. Data using the CODOX-M/IVAC regimen in HIV positive adults with Burkitt lymphoma suggests its feasibility in these patients [33 – 37]. The AIDS Malignancy Consortium reported on 34 patients treated with CODOX-M/IVAC plus rituximab [36, 37]. With a median age of 42 years and a CD4 count of 195/uL, 20 patients

had severe myelosuppression and 14 had severe infections complicating therapy [37]. With one treatment-related death, the 1-year progression-free survival was 69% and overall survival was 72% [37].

Progress on DA-EPOCH-R

Utilizing infusional etoposide, vincristine and doxorubicin, the dose-adjusted EPOCH regimen combine with rituximab appears to provide excellent results in a less intensive manner [36, 37]. A prospective trail reported on 19 patients treated with DA-EPOCH-R and 11 patients with HIV-related BL treated with a short course of EPOCH with dose intensive rituximab [37]. After more than 6years of f/u in both groups, the rate of freedom from disease progression were 95% and 100% in the HIV negative and HIV positive cohorts respectively [37]. While designed to achieve an absolute neutrophil count of <500 cells per cubic milliliter, only 22% of DA-EPOCH-R cycles were complicated by febrile neutropenia [35 -37]. Further, severe gastrointestinal events were rare and grade 3 or 4 sensory neuropathy occurred in 17% of patients (Table 3) [36, 37].

This Cancer and Leukemia Group B developed regimen is a dose-intensive short-duration treatment plan lasting 18 weeks in duration. Following a seven-day cycle of cyclophosphamide and prednisone, patients receive alternating cycles of ifosfamide, methotrexate, vincristine, cytarabine, etoposide, dexamethasone with cyclophosphamide, methotrexate, vincristine, doxorubicin, and dexamethasone [30, 37]. The inclusion of prophylactic cranial radiation to high-risk individuals and the initially observed neurologic side effects may partially account for its limited use [37].

Largely studied in children and adolescents, this dose-intense regimen divides patients into four different risk categories, allocating the most intense and toxic treatment to patients with higher risk disease [31, 32, 37]. The prognostic groups are based on whether the disease has been surgically resected, stage, LDH, leukemic presentation, and central nervous system (CNS) [31, 32, 37].

Based on risk group, patients received two to six cycles of chemotherapy. For all patients except those with completely resected disease, treatment was preceded by a less intense prophase cycle intended to improve the patient's performance status [30-32, 37]. More than 500 patients were investigated on this protocol, demonstrating excellent event-free survival rates, further, the demonstrated that for patients with limited stage disease, the high-dose methotrexate dose and infusion could be reduced without compromising outcomes [31, 37].

Table 3. In CALGB 9251 [36]

Cycle 1
Cyclophosphamide 200 mg/m2IV on days 1-5
Prednisone 60 mg/m2orally in days 1-7
Cycles 2, 4 and 6
Ifosfamide 800 mg/m2IV od days 1-5 with mesna uroprotection
Methotrexate150 mg/m^2 IV over 30 min, then 1.35 g/m2IV over 23.5 hrs
Leucovorin rescue begins 36 hours from the start of the methotrexate infusion
Vincristine 2 mg IV on day 1
Cytarabine150 mg/m2on days 4 and 5
Etoposide80 mg/m^2 IV on days 4 and 5
Dexamethasone 10 mg/m2orally on days 1-5
Cycles 3, 5 and 7
Cyclophosphamide200 mg/m2IV on days 1-5
Methotrexate150 mg/m^2 IV over 30 min, then 1.35 g/m2 IV over 23.5 hrs Leucovorin rescue begins 36 hours from the start of the methotrexate infusion.
Vincristine2 mg IV on day 1
Doxorubicin 25 mg/m^2IV on days 4 and 5
Dexamethasone 10 mg/m2orally on days 1-5
Intrathecal prophylaxiswith Cycles 2-7
Methotrexate15 mg IT on day 1
Cytarabine40 mg IT on day 1
Hydrocortisone50 mg IT on day 1
Cranial irradiation: 2400 cGy administered in 12 fractions after Cycle 7 was completed, but only for patients who presented with bone marrow disease

Table 4. In Hyper-CVAD alternating with MA [36]

Hyper-CVAD (cycles 1, 3, 5, 7)
Cyclophosphamide300 mg/m2IV every 12 hours on days 1-3 (6 doses) with mesna uropotection
Vincristtine2 mg IV on days 4 and 11
Doxorubicin50 mg/m2IV over 24 hours on day 4
Dexamethasone 40 mg daily on days 1-4 and 11-14
Rituximab 375 mg/m2IV on days 1 and 11(cycles 1 and 3)
MA (cycles 2, 4, 6, 8)
Methotrexate1gm/m2IV over 24 hours on day 1
Leucovorin rescue begins 24 hours from the start of the methotrexate infusion.
Cytarabine3gm/m2IV every 12 hours on days 2and 3 (4 doses) (For patients older than 60 years, 1gm/m^2)
Rituximab 375 mg/m2IV on days 2and 8(cycles 2and 4)
Granulocyte colony-stimulating factor started 24 hours after chemotherapy completion until the absolute neutrophil count is > 3.0x109/L
Intrathecal prophylaxis:
Methotrexate 12 mg IT on day 2
Cytarabine 100 mg IT on day 7

Similar to the Berlin-Frankfurt-Munich (BFM) protocol, LMB 96 protocol was developed to bhe used in children and adolescents. It is a dose-intense chemotherapy regimen where patients are stratified into therapy groups based on surgical resection of disease, CNS involvement, and degree of bone marrow involvement [36, 37]. This regimen also demonstrated excellent results in these younger patients and the ability to achieve comparable outcomes across risk groups by using prephase treatment, tailoring the therapy intensity based on above factors and aggressively prophylaxing/treating patients for CNS disease (Table 4) [31, 32, 36, 37]. As a result, it has been hailed as yielding high survival rates in Burkitt's lymphoma (BL) and diffuse large cell lymphoma (DLCL) in children, as well as in primary cerebral DLCL (PCL) of adults [31, 32, 36, 37].

The hyper-CVAD regimen was initially developed for patients with acute lymphoblastic leukemia but has been evaluated in BL.

Hyperfractionated cyclophosphamide, vincristine, doxorubicin, and dexamethasone is alternated with high dose methotrexate and cytarabine for 8 cycles. Results with and without rituximab have been encouraging, albeit in a more heterogeneous population than CODOX-M/IVAC was evaluated in.

With regards to the optimal up front treatment regimen, comparative studies are not available. Usually, younger patients have been treated with the CODOX-M/IVAC protocol. Among the published variations on the regimen, all are reasonable options with comparable efficacy and toxicity. In addition, rituximab has been included with first-line treatment. Likewise, patients with HIV-associated disease have been typically treated in similar manner. The NCI-generated results using DA-EPOCH-R suggest that excellent outcomes may be obtained with less intensive infusional therapy. However, this regimen requires treating physicians to adjust the doxorubicin, etoposide and cyclophosphamide doses based on neutrophil and platelet nadirs with each cycle. For older patients or those unable to tolerate a short-course, dose-intensive regimen, the dose-adjusted EPOCH-R regimen may provide the best risk to benefit ratio for this population. Standard RCHOP should be considered as being palliative in this population.

Autologous stem cell transplantation has been evaluated as a consolidative strategy after patients have received initial therapy. While data are limited, results suggest comparable outcomes to those obtained with the short –course regimens listed above.

Few options exist for patients who relapse after initial therapy. Typical salvage regimens used in diffuse large B-cell lymphoma such as ICE (ifosfamide, carboplatin, etoposide) or DHAP (dexamethasone, cytarabine, cisplatin) can at times be used to bridge patients to either autologous or allogeneic stem cell transplantation.

Post-chemotherapy supportive care is critical given the dose intensity and subsequent side effects associated with standard treatment regimens. As such, close outpatient follow-up to monitor side effects and transfusion requirements is needed. Patients require appropriate inpatients resources and staff experienced in chemotherapy administration and their respective side effects. Most notably is the sophistication involved in the use of IV high-dose methotrexate. Patients require pre-treatment hydration and alkalinization, monitoring urine pH, renal and hepatic function, rapid turnaround in methotrexate levels, attention to leucovorin rescue, and availability of carboxypeptidase in rare circumstances.

Prevention and management of tumor lysis syndrome typically includes aggressive intravenous hydration and the urate oxidase, rasburicase. In the event of renal failure from uric acid nephropathy, management may include hemodialysis [28, 29, 38]. Additionally, granulocyte colony-stimulating factor support as well as antibacterial, antiviral and antifungal prophylaxis are routinely administered [29, 38].

Burkitt lymphoma is rapidly progressive and universally fatal in the absence of therapy, in patients able to tolerate a dose-intensive chemotherapy program, timely initiation and completion of therapy can result in long-term survival. While most patients will initially respond to treatment, progression-free and overall survival rate in adults have not matched outcomes in younger patients. Using the CODOX-M/IVAC regimen, investigators have reported two-year overall survival ranging from 67-92%. At five years, CLGB 9251 resulted in 52% of patients being alive and in complete remission. Three-year overall survival for hyper-CVAF has ranged from 49-89% [38]. Six-year overall survival for DA-EPOCH-R has been reported to be 100%, albeit in 19 patients have a median age of 33 years [38]. For patients who relapse after initial therapy, salvage options should be considered palliative given few patients achieving long-term survival [38].

Other factors to consider in BL management are as follows:

Situation of When a Patient Is Too Ill to Receive Chemotherapy

Due to the rapidly progressive nature of BL, patients may present with evidence of end-organ dysfunction or a poor performance status secondary to lymphoma. Based on experience with other malignancies, medical professionals and intensive care unit staff may assume that the patient isn't able to tolerate chemotherapy [38, 39]. Patients with BL may experience a rapid improvement in function with appropriate treatment.

It has been reported that some clinical trial experience have demonstrated that temporizing measures such as fractionated cyclophosphamide or a single cycle of CHOP chemotherapy can allow for time to confirm the diagnosis and improve a patient's performance status without compromising the patients' chance of cure [7, 9, 39]. Measures such as these may also be used in the critically ill patients to optimize organ function prior to starting a dose-intensive regimen [37-39].

When There Is a Lack of Referral to a Specialist/Secondary/Tertiary Care Unit

Given the need for close monitoring of patients during therapy, the use of high-dose methotrexate, and aggressive tumor lysis prophylaxis, most patients should be treated by staff experienced in managing BL [28, 29, 39]. As such, clinical intuition and a prompt diagnosis are important to allow for transfer of the patient's care to a specialist unit for efficient and effective management [40, 41]. Consequently, lack of timely referral of patient care to a specialist unit or tertiary care center may result in worst outcome for the patient.

Normally functioning as a transcription regulator, constitutive overexpression of the MYC oncogene plays a primary role in the pathogenesis of BL [7-9, 39]. While c-MYC expression is not uncommon in other malignancies, this typically represents a secondary alternation occurring in the setting of clonal evolution [7-10, 39]. In BL, c-MYC overexpression typically results from a chromosomal translocation between the c-MYC oncogene on the long arm of chromosome 8 and either the Ig heavy chain gene on chromosome 22. As a result of the MYC oncogene juxtaposing with one of the immunoglobulin gene loci, the c-MYC allele is expressed constitutively and cell cycle control is lost [7-9, 39].

Next-generation sequencing has revealed a number of diverse genetic abnormalities contributing to the pathogenesis of BL [5-9, 12, 15, 39]. Among the most common include recurrent silencing mutations in the tumor suppressor gene ID3 leading to constitutive activation of the transcription factor TCF-3 [5-9, 12, 15, 39], thus promoting cell-cycle progression through CCND3 [9, 12, 15, 39].

In addition, more poorly understood genetic lesions simultaneously inhibit apoptosis [12, 15, 39]. One such mechanism includes EBV, the genome of which in contained in tumor cell nuclei in some cases, mostly commonly in endemic and HIV related disease [19, 39]. This accounts for the majority of endemic African Burkitt lymphomas where it is hypothesized that malaria cases B-cell hyperplasia facilitating disease genesis in the setting of widespread EBV [7-9, 19, 39]. This explanation does not account for the majority of cases in developed countries where10-20% of cases are EVB-related [12, 15, 39].

The rapid nature of disease presentation and progression is the most salient feature obtained in patient's history. Insidious non-specific symptoms over a prolonged time course are uncommon [19, 39]. Inquiring about risk factors for HIV may be helpful in identifying immunodeficiency-related disease [19, 39]. Patients may have systemic complaints or B symptoms defined as fever of more than 38°C, weight loss of more than 10% of body weight, or the presence of drenching night sweats [3, 7-9, 19, 39].

Enlarged lymphadenopathy, abdominal masses, or organomegaly may be palpable on physical exam [40]. In conjunction, a rapidly declining performance status may be evident [3, 39, 40].

Analysis to identify overexpression of BCL-2, most commonly due to the t(14;18) translocation, is identified in a small number of cases by routine karyotype analysis or FISH [5, 7-9, 41]. More rarely, a translocation involving the BCL-6 gene on chromosome 3q27 may be identified. These so-called "double hit" lymphomas have an extremely poor prognosis with a median overall survival reported 2.5 months in one series [40, 41].

Updates on Prognosis of BL

The current cure rate of BL is in the order of 80-90% thanks to a difficult, but relatively short treatment that is without long term sequelae [3, 7-9, 30-41]. The patient's outcome depends on the stage of BL at diagnosis [39, 41]. It has been noted that the outlook is usually worse in adults over the age of 40, but treatment for adults has improved in recent years [41]. The outlook is poor in people who have HIV, but it is significantly better in people whose cancer has not spread to other parts of the body [40, 41].

CONCLUSION

BL is a rare form of malignant aggressive mature B-cell NHL. Management of BL should be carried out in a specialist oncology/ hematology centers. Treatment is with a few months of intensive chemotherapy. The efficacy of rituximab has not yet been proven but it is the subject of several clinical trials. BL constitutes a therapeutic emergency. In addition, at diagnosis, about 70% of patients are in the advance stages of the disease. Hence, BL is considered to be a highly aggressive tumor. Involvement of the bone marrow and CNS tumor size >10 cm diameter, and elevated serum LDH are considered poor prognostic factors. Again, response to intensive combination chemotherapy with complete remission reaches 90% in early stages and 60–80% in advanced stages of the disease. Allogenic bone marrow transplantation has been given to patients not responding to chemotherapy. The key to curing the disease is a combination of rapid and individualized management (particularly adapted to the frequent metabolic problems that occur at the start of treatment) and appropriate anti-tumor treatment. Future work will involve investigating more on, and providing further data on the better understanding of the EBV influences on the genesis of the endemic form of BL, with a view of developing guidelines for better diagnosis and management of BL, including giving insights to more research and innovations for providing improved outcomes and prognosis for suffers of the disease.

REFERENCES

[1] https://www.cancer.ca/en/cancer-information/cancer-type/non-hodgkin-lymphoma/non-hodgkin-lymphoma/more-types-of-nhl/burkitt-lymphoma/?region=on. Accessed on May 16 2021.

[2] Hummel, M., Bentink, S. & Bergenr, H. (2006). A biologic definition of Burkitt's lymphoma from transcriptional and genomic profiling. *N Engl J Med.*, *354*, 2419-2430.

[3] Molyneux, E. M., Rochfrod, R., Griffin, B., Newton, R., Jackson, G., Menon, G., et al. (2012). Burkitt's lymphoma. *Lancet.*, 2012 Mar 31. *379* (9822), 1234-44.

[4] Gong, J. Z., Stenzel, T. T., Bennett, E. R., et al. (2003). Burkitt lymphoma arising in organ transplant recipients: a clinicopathologic study of five case. *Am J Surg Pathol.*, *27*(6), 818-27.

[5] Dave, S. S., Fu, K. & Wright, G. W. (2006). Molecular diagnosis of Burkitt's lymphoma. *N Engl J Med.*, *354*, 2431-2442.

[6] *Burkitt Lymphoma*: https://www.orpha.net/consor/cgi-bin/OC_Exp.php?Lng=GB&Expert=543 Accessed on May 16 2021.

[7] Dang, C. V., Resar, L. M., Emison, E., et al. Function of the c-Myc oncogenic transcription factor. *Exp Cell Res.*, Nov 25, *253*(1), 63-77.

[8] Dang, C. V. V., O'Donnell, K. A. & Juopperi, T. (2005). The great MYC escape in tumorigenesis. *Cancer Cell*, *8*(3), 177-8.

[9] Coller, H. A., Grandori, C., Tamayo, P., et al. (2000). Expression analysis with oligonucleotide microarrays reveals that MYC regulates genes involved in growth, cell cycle, signaling, and adhesion. *Proc Natl Acad Sci U S A*, *97*(7), 3260-5.

[10] Burkitt, D. P. (1972). Classics in oncology. A sarcoma involving the jaws in African children. *CA Cancer J Clin.*, 1972 Nov-Dec., *22*(6), 345-55.

[11] Burkitt, D. & O'Conor, G. T. (1961). Malignant lymphoma in African children. I. A clinical syndrome. *Cancer*, *14*, 258-69.

[12] Magrath, I. T. (1991). African Burkitt's lymphoma. History, biology, clinical features, and treatment. *Am J Pediatr Hematol Oncol.*, *13*(2), 222-46.

[13] Epstein, M. A., Achong, B. G. & Barr, Y. M. (1964). Virus particles in cultured lymphoblasts from Burkitt's lymphoma. *Lancet*, *1*(7335), 702-3.

[14] World Health Organization classification of Burkitt Lymphoma. (2021) at: https://www.who.int/. Accessed on May 16 2021.

[15] Magrath, I. (1990). The pathogenesis of Burkitt's lymphoma. *Adv Cancer Res.*, *55*, 133-270.

[16] Ferry, J. A. (2006). Burkitt's lymphoma: clinicopathologic features and differential diagnosis. *Oncologist*, *11*(4), 375-83.

[17] De Falco, G., Antonicelli, G., Onnis, A., Lazzi, S., Bellan, C. & Leoncini, L. (2009). Role of EBV in microRNA dysregulation in Burkitt lymphoma. *Semin Cancer Biol.*, *19*(6), 401-6.

[18] Thorley-Lawson, D. A. & Allday, M. J. (2008). The curious case of the tumour virus: 50 years of Burkitt's lymphoma. *Nat Rev Microbiol*, *6*(12), 913-24.

[19] Davi, F., Delecluse, H. J., Guiet, P., et al. (1998). Burkitt-like lymphomas in AIDS patients: characterization within a series of 103 human immunodeficiency virus-associated non-Hodgkin's lymphomas. Burkitt's Lymphoma Study Group. *J Clin Oncol.*, *16*(12), 3788-95.

[20] Cardy, H. A., Sharp, L. & Little, J. (2001). Burkitt's lymphoma: a review of the epidemiology. *Kuwait Med J.*, *33*, 293-306.

[21] Makata, A. M., Toriyama, K., Kamidigo, N. O., Eto, H. & Itakura, H. (1996). The pattern of pediatric solid malignant tumors in western Kenya, east Africa, 1979-1994: an analysis based on histopathologic study. *Am J Trop Med Hyg.*, *54*(4), 343-7.

[22] Swerdlow, S. H., et al. (2008). *WHO Classification of Tumours of Haematopoietic and Lymphoid Tissues.* 4th Edition. Lyon, France: International Agency for Research on Cancer.

[23] https://www.cancertherapyadvisor.com/home/decision-support-in-medicine/hematology/burkitt-lymphoma-2/. Accessed on May 16 2021.

[24] https://radiopaedia.org/articles/ann-arbor-staging-system. Accessed on May 16 2021.

[25] Magrath, I., Adde, M., Shad, A., et al. (1996). Adults and children with small non-cleaved-cell lymphoma have a similar excellent outcome when treated with the same chemotherapy regimen. *J Clin Oncol.*, *14*(3), 925-34.

[26] Ferry, J. A. (2006). Burkitt's lymphoma: clinicopathologic features and differential diagnosis. *Onclogist.*, *11*(4), 375-83.

[27] Rizzieri, D. A., Johnson, J. L. & Niedzwiecki, D. (2004). Intensive chemotherapy with and without cranial radiation for Burkitt leukemia and lymphoma: final results of Cancer and leukemia Group B Study 9251. *Cancer.*, vol. *100*, pp. 1438-1448.

[28] Cario, M. S. & Bishop, M. (2004). Tumour lysis syndrome: new therapeutic strategies and classification. *Br J Haematol.*, *127*(1), 3-11.

[29] Jones, G. L., et al. (2015). Guidelines for the management of tumour lysis syndrome in adults and children with haematological malignancies on behalf of the British Committee for Standards in Haematology. *Br J Haematol.*, *169*(5), 661-71.

[30] Dunleavy, K., Piitaluga, S. & Shovlin, N. (2013). Low-Intensity Therapy in Adults with Burkitt's Lymphoma. *N Engl J Med.*, *369*, 1915-25.

[31] Dozzo, M., Carobolante, F., Donisi, P. M., Scattolin, A., Maino, E., Sancetta, R., Viero, P. & Bassan, R. (2007). *Burkitt lymphoma in adolescents and young adults: management challenges, Adolesc Health Med Ther.*, *8*, 11-29.

[32] Linch, D. C. (2012). Burkitt lymphoma in adults. *Br J Haematol.*, *156*(6), 693-703.

[33] Mead, G. M., Sydes, M. R. & Walewski, J. (2002). An international evaluation of CODOX-M and CODOX-M alternating with IVAC in adults Burkitt's lymphoma: results of United Kingdom Lymphoma Group LY06 study. *Ann Oncol.*, *13*, 1264-1274.

[34] Noy, A., Lee, J. Y. & Cesarman, E. (2015). AMC 048: modified CODOX-M/IVAC-rituximab is an effective HIV-associated Burkitt lymphoma. *Blood.*, *126*, 160-6.

[35] Evens, A. M., Carson, K. R. & Kolesar, K. (2013). A multicentre phase II study incorporating high-dose rituximab and liposomal doxorubicin into CODOX-M/IVAC regimen for untreated Burkitt's lymphoma. *Annals of Oncology*, *24*, 3076-81.

[36] Mead, G. M., Barrans, S. L. & Qian, W. (2008). A prospective clinicopathologic study of dose-modified CODOX-M/IVAC in patients with sporadic Burkitt lymphoma defined using cytogenetic and immunophenotypic criteria (MRC/NCRILY10 trial). *Blood*, *112*, 2248-2260.

[37] Davi, F., Delecluse, H. J., Guiet, P., et al. (1998). Burkitt-like lymphomas in AIDS patients: characterization within a series of 103 human immunodeficiency virus-associated non-Hodgkin's lymphomas. Burkitt's Lymphoma Study Group. *J Clin Oncol.*, *16*(12), 3788-95.

[38] Thomas, D. A., Faderl, S. & O'Brien, S. (2006). Chemoimmunotherapy with hyper-CVAD plus rituximab for treatment of adult Burkitt and Burkitt-type lymphoma or acute lymphoblastic leukemia. *Cancer ol.*, *106*, 1569-1580.

[39] Kelly, J. L., Toothaker, S. R. & Ciminello, L. (2009). Outcomes of patients with Burkitt lymphoma older than age 40 treated with intensive chemotherapeutic regimes. *Clin Lymphoma Myeloma*, *9*, 307-310.

[40] Lacasce, A., Howard, O. & Lib, S. (2003). Modified Magrath regimens for adults with Burkitt and Burkitt like lymphomas: preserved efficacy with decreased toxicity. *Leuk Lymphoma*, *45*, 761-7.

[41] Magrath, I., Adde, M. & Shad, A. (1996). Adults and children with small non-cleaved-cell lymphoma have a similar excellent outcome when treated with the same chemotherapy regimen. *JCO*, *14*, 925-34.

INDEX

A

B

E

F

G

H

N

O

P

R

S

T

U

V

W

Y